CROSS-CULTURAL ANXIETY

THE SERIES IN CLINICAL AND COMMUNITY PSYCHOLOGY

CONSULTING EDITORS
Charles D. Spielberger and Irwin G. Sarason

IN PREPARATION

CROSS-CULTURAL ANXIETY

ANXIETY

Volume 4

Edited by
Charles D. Spielberger
University of South Florida

Rogelio Diaz-Guerrero
National University of Mexico

Guest Editor
Jan Strelau
University of Warsaw

● HEMISPHERE PUBLISHING CORPORATION
A member of the Taylor & Francis Group

New York   Washington   Philadelphia   London

CROSS-CULTURAL ANXIETY: Volume 4

1 2 3 4 5 6 7 8 9 0   BRBR   9 8 7 6 5 4 3 2 1 0

This book was set in Times Roman by Hemisphere Publishing Corporation. The editors were Deena Williams Newman and Kathleen Porta; the production supervisor was Peggy M. Rote; and the typesetter was Phoebe Carter. Cover design by Sharon M. DePass.
Printing and binding by Braun-Brumfield, Inc.

A CIP catalog record for this book is available from the British Library.

Library of Congress Cataloging-in-Publication Data

(Revised for vol. 2)
Main entry under title:

Cross-cultural anxiety.

   (The series in clinical and community psychology,
0146-0846)
   Vol 1: "Based on a symposium at the XVth
Interamerican Congress of Psychology, Bogotá, Colombia,
in December, 1974"
   Vol. 4: Washington: Hemisphere Pub.
   Includes bibliographies and indexes.
   1. Anxiety—Cross cultural studies—Congresses.
I. Spielberger, Charles Donald, date.   II. Díaz
Guerrero, Rogelio.   III. Series.
BF575.A6C76   152.4   76-28389
ISBN 0-89116-940-7
ISSN 0146-0846

Contents

Contributors

JAMES C. BARTLETT, University of Texas at Dallas, USA
JOSÉ J. BAUERMEISTER, University of Puerto Rico, Río Piedras, Puerto Rico
MIRIAM BEN-RAFAEL, Geha Psychiatric Hospital, Petach-Tigra, Israel
JERI BENSON, University of Maryland, College Park, MD, USA
ANGELA M. B. BIAGGO, Universidade Federal do Rio Grande do Sul, Brazil
PETR BLAHUS, Charles University, Prague, Czechoslovakia
JOHN BREBNER, University of Adelaide, Australia
ROGELIO DIAZ-GUERRERO, National University of Mexico, Mexico City, Mexico
DOMINGO E. GÓMEZ-FERNÁNDEZ, University of Santiago de Compostela, Spain
HANA GILAIE, Tel Aviv University, Israel
DIETER HACKFORT, Institut für Sport und Sportwissenschaft, University of Heidelberg,
    Federal Republic of Germany
KNUT A. HAGTVET, University of Bergen, Norway
KJELL HASETH, University of Oslo, Norway
JOHN J. HEDL, JR., University of Texas at Dallas, USA
FRANTISEK MAN, Pedagogical Faculty, Ceské Budéjovice, Czechoslovakia
IVAN G. PASPALANOV, University of Sofia, Bulgaria
PHILIP A. SAIGH, City University of New York, USA
PETER SCHULZ, University of Trier, Federal Republic of Germany
CHARLES D. SPIELBERGER, University of South Florida, Tampa, FL, USA
YONA TEICHMAN, Tel Aviv University, Israel
ELIZABETH TIPPETS, University of Maryland, College Park, MD, USA
MILDRED VERA, University of Puerto Rico, Río Piedras, Puerto Rico
RANIER WIELAND-ECKELMAN, Bergisch Universität-Gesamthochschule—Wuppertal,
    Federal Republic of Germany
KAZIMIERZ WRZESNIEWSKI, Warsaw Medical Academy, Warsaw, Poland

Preface

Since the publication some 14 years ago of the first volume in this series, cross-cultural research on anxiety has greatly accelerated and the quality of the studies in this field has steadily improved. Moreover, the theoretical formulations that have guided the research and the methodology of the investigations have become evermore sophisticated. This research has also been stimulated by and has benefited from international conferences that have occurred with increasing frequency.

Volume 4 of this continuing series is composed of a number of papers that were initially presented at an international conference on Stress and Anxiety held in Rynia, Poland, in September 1983. Sponsored by the Polish Academy of Sciences and the Faculty of Psychology at the University of Warsaw, the conference in Poland attracted more than 60 participants from 15 countries. The conference papers were subsequently revised and expanded, and additional chapters were contributed by investigators who were actively engaged in cross-cultural research on anxiety and its effects on behavior. Professor Jan Strelau of the University of Warsaw, who was primarily responsible for organizing the Rynia conference, served as Guest Editor of this volume.

The contents of this volume are divided into three major parts. It is perhaps significant to note that the authors of the six chapters that constitute Part I report research findings from four continents and six different countries. These studies describe the impact on anxiety of a variety of stressful circumstances and a large number of individual difference variables in research on children, adults, and the elderly. Although the importance of the experience of anxiety as an internal emotional state has been increasingly recognized, there is still a great deal of controversy with regard to the essential nature of anxiety and its effects on behavior.

The five chapters in Part II of this volume examine the relation of anxiety to various forms of coping behavior, and how anxiety influences perception, cognition, and a variety of behavioral performance measures. Specific topics that are considered include the effects of situational stress and individual differences in anxiety proneness on coping style, memory, comprehension, and sports-related performance.

The research reported in the final section is concerned primarily with the construction and validation of measures of anxiety for use in cross-cultural research. Research findings are reported on the assessment of state, trait, and test anxiety in five different countries: Brazil, Czechoslovakia, Norway, Spain, and the United States. The research on state and trait anxiety in Brazil, Norway, and Spain not only reveals a number of interesting similarities, but also some striking cultural differences. The cross-cultural consistency of the Worry and Emotionality factors identified in research on test anxiety in Czechslovakia and the United States is also especially impressive.

The contents of this book will be of interest to educators and behavioral and medical scientists who are concerned with cross-cultural research on stress and anxiety, human personality and abnormal behavior, and the reduction of anxiety in the treatment and rehabilitation of psychiatric and medical patients. The research findings will also provide important information for psychologists and educators interested in the effects of anxiety on human performance, and for mental health specialists engaged in clinical practice, especially those who work with bilingual clients and patients who come from different cultures.

For their dedicated contributions to planning and coordinating the conference in Poland, we express our gratitude to Prorektor Professor Stanislaw Kaluzynski, and to the faculty and graduate students of the Department of Psychology of Individual Differences at the University of Warsaw. We also thank Tatiana Klonowicz and Tytus Sosnowski of the University of Warsaw and Susan Krasner, Richard Rickman, and Veronica Clement of the University of South Florida for their invaluable contributions in reviewing the manuscripts. Finally, we express our appreciation to Virginia Berch for her expert technical and clerical assistance in preparing the manuscript for publication.

Charles D. Spielberger
Rogelio Diaz-Guerrero
Jan Strelau

I

STRESS AND ANXIETY

1

Gender and Social Class Determinants of Anxiety in the Mexican Culture

Rogelio Diaz-Guerrero
National University of Mexico

Anxiety is a critical and universal human phenomenon. In the past 20 years, significant advances have been made on its reliable and valid measurement for groups of different ages, social classes, and cultures. This progress would not have been possible without the development of a theory sensitive to the characteristics of human anxiety and the availability of an instrument of measurement that is isomorphic with the theory and universally reliable in its content.

Through a painstaking process, C. D. Spielberger (1966, 1972, 1979) and his students have developed a theoretical conception that recognizes two critical facets of anxiety, that is, anxiety as a generalized trait (anxiety proneness) and anxiety as an emotional state or response evoked by situational stressors that are perceived as threatening. The State–Trait Anxiety Inventory (STAI) was constructed to measure these two facets of anxiety (Spielberger, Gorsuch, & Lushene, 1970). Careful translations and psychometric adaptations of the STAI have stimulated a large number of studies in the United States and in many different cultures (Spielberger & Diaz-Guerrero, 1976, 1983, 1986).

An important area of anxiety research that has been little probed to date relates to the types of stresses that are specifically threatening for men and women, and for persons of different ages, social classes, or cultures. Magnusson, Stattin, and Iwawaki (1983) have criticized the use of the trait measurement model in cross-cultural research because this model fails to account for situational variation in anxiety behavior. Using a cross-cultural, quasi-experimental design, these investigators obtained reports of physiological and emotional reactions to 17 hypothetical anxiety-provoking situations. Although they found a number of gender and cross-cultural differences for Swedish and Japanese adolescents, they noted the limitations in the self-report techniques used in their study that were based on merely hypothetical anxiety-provoking situations rather than real-life stressors.

It is difficult to design stressful real-life stimulus situations that are universally perceived as threatening and that still show differential threat value across sex and social class. It would be even more difficult to expose large groups of subjects, one by one, to a variety of stressful situations.[1] The methodological alternative used in this study was to expose Mexican adolescents to concepts that are repre-

---

[1]To follow this social psychological experimental approach would require a great deal of work, with the following steps: (a) Operationally define each concept (e.g., sadness); (b) develop a laboratory strategy to provoke sadness in each subject; (c) measure, by an ad hoc questionnaire, the degree of

sentative of potentially threatening stressors, to measure the reaction to these concepts with a reliable measure of subjective meaning (Osgood's semantic differential), and to ascertain the relation of these subjective judgments to anxiety proneness.

I investigated sources of anxiety within the Mexican culture as a function of
gender and social class. The major questions to be answered were as follows:
which of the threatening concepts were universally related in cognition to greater
anxiety proneness, and which were sex or class specific? The 20 clinically critical
anxiety-provoking concepts, developed by Jose Lichtszajn and myself (Diaz-
Guerrero, Lichtszajn & Reyes-Lagunes, 1979; Lichtszajn, 1979), were aggression, cancer, crime, death, drunkenness, divorce, fear, funeral, hunger, insult to
the mother, madness, myself, life, old age, pain, sadness, separation from family,
separation from school, sickness, and suicide. The semantic differential technique
was used to rate each concept according to the three subjective meaning factors
described by Osgood, Suci, and Tannenbaum (1957): evaluation, potency, and
activity. A scale to measure familiarity with the concepts was added to assess this
additional possible source of stress and anxiety.

This study strives to determine important sources of threat and anxiety for
adolescents in the Mexican culture, along with the subcultural variance attributable
to sex and social class. Given the correlational research design, it would be equally
appropriate to interpret the findings as indicating that the more anxiety-prone persons (higher trait anxiety score) were more threatened by the subjective meaning
of certain concepts, or that those who were threatened experienced anxiety more
frequently. The former approach to interpretation, which follows from my theory
that the cultural ecosystem is an indispensable mediator of personality development (Diaz-Guerrero, 1979, 1980; Diaz-Guerrero & Castillo Vales, 1981), is followed in this study. It is further assumed that the ecosystem can be assessed by
using scales that measure historic-sociocultural premises (Diaz-Guerrero, 1982a,
1986a, 1986b).

SOURCES OF ANXIETY
IN MEXICAN ADOLESCENTS

The participants were 200 junior high school students, aged 14–16 years old,
attending state and private schools in Mexico City. The sample contained equal
numbers of male and female students from the upper-lower and upper-middle social
classes. Socioeconomic level was based on occupation and education, using an index
developed for Mexico by Calatayud, Reyes-Lagunes, Avila, and Diaz-Guerrero
(1974). The upper-lower-class groups consisted of children from families of skilled
workers or those who had occupations with similar levels of education and income.
The upper-middle-class groups included children whose fathers were professional
men or who had occupations that were comparable in education and income.

The Pancultural Spanish Semantic Differential Scale (Diaz-Guerrero & Salas,

---

sadness in each subject; (d) identify subjects high and low in sadness; (e) have each subject respond to
Spielberger's STAI Trait Anxiety scale. An analysis of variance with two levels of sadness should then
show what is reported later, for instance that lower class men have relatively greater anxiety related to
sadness. However, obtaining results for the 20 concepts that are investigated in this study would
demand 20 experiments!

1975; Osgood, May, & Myron, 1975) was used to evaluate the critical clinical concepts. It was administered to groups of students in their natural classrooms, with the consent of the students and their teachers and principals. Immediately before judging the critical clinical concepts, the students completed the Trait Anxiety Scale of the *Inventario de Ansiedad, Rasgo y Estado* (IDARE), the Spanish language form of the STAI (Spielberger & Diaz-Guerrero, 1975). Table 1 reports the means and standard deviations of the scores on Spielberger's Trait Anxiety Scale for the four groups of students, who did not differ significantly in trait anxiety. Thus, the students in this population of adolescents were highly homogeneous in anxiety proneness.

The subjective appraisal of four of the critical concepts (fear, funeral, separation from family, suicide) did not pose a significant threat to this adolescent population. The findings for the remaining 16 concepts, reported in Table 2, are highly complex and heterogeneous. For the total group, 11 concepts were significant sources of anxiety: low self-evaluation (myself), low evaluation of life, high activity related to insult to the mother, greater familiarity with separation from school, and higher potency for drunkenness, pain, sickness, aggression, crime, death, and sadness.

Social class, gender, and the combination of these variables produced a number of specific results. High potency associated with drunkenness, which was threatening to the entire sample of adolescents, was more threatening for the lower-class students. For the lower-class students, a positive (actually less negative) evaluation of pain and separation from school was associated with higher trait anxiety, and higher perceived activity for life and hunger was more threatening than for upper-middle-class students. Sadness, which was perceived as the greatest threat for the entire sample, was much more potent for lower-class than for middle-class students, particularly for the boys. The middle-class students perceived the power of aggression as more threatening. They also reported greater anxiety with familiarity with the concepts of separation from school and cancer and a lower evaluation of life and old age.

Typical sources of anxiety for the girls, in contrast to the boys, was a lower perceived activity of the self and higher perceived activity of separation from school. The boys reported the potency of pain, sickness, madness, and sadness as being more threatening than did the girls. Boys also reported greater anxiety about their familiarity with separation from school.

The specificity of the sources of threat was greatest when the combined effects of gender and social class were evaluated. Lower-class boys must be distinguished from the other groups; for them, 13 of the 20 critical concepts were perceived as threatening, compared with only 3 for the upper-middle-class boys, 8 for the upper-middle-class girls, and 6 for the lower-class girls. In most cases, this sub-

Table 1 Means and Standard Deviations in Trait Anxiety by Sex and Social Class

Groups	M	SD
Upper-lower-class men	38.4	7.28
Upper-middle-class men	39.1	7.21
Upper-lower-class women	39.1	6.58
Upper-middle-class women	39.2	7.54

Table 2 The Relation of Threatening Concepts to Anxiety Trait in Mexico (Spielberger's Anxiety Trait)

Concepts	Boys		Girls		All boys	All girls	Upper lower class	Upper middle class	Total group
	Upper lower class	Upper middle class	Upper lower class	Upper middle class					
Insult to the mother E	.30*	.01	-.02	-.12					
Insult to the mother A	.05	.10	.36*	.10					.15*
Insult to the mother F	.32*	-.15	-.08	-.07					
Drunkenness P	.29*	.23	.32*	.20			.31***		.26***
Myself E	-.37**	-.07	-.07	-.27					
Myself P	.27	.03	-.40**	.06					-.20**
Myself A	.16	.06	-.23	-.31*					
Pain E	.37**	-.14	.12	-.09		-.27**			.16*
Pain P	.25	.34*	.03	.03	.30**		.25**		
Sickness E	-.01	-.30*	-.05	.05					
Sickness P	.42**	.14	-.04	.11	.28**				.16*
Sickness A	.49***	.03	.04	-.05					
Aggression P	.21	.14	-.07	.28*				.21*	.14*
Life E	-.11	-.19	-.21	-.22			.24*	-.21*	-.18**
Life A	.33*	-.09	.14	-.03			.21*		
Separation from school E	.29*	.09	.13	-.13					
Separation from school P	.12	.01	-.23	.40**					
Separation from school A	.03	-.05	.26	.38**		.32**			
Separation from school F	.19	.38**	-.07	.12	.29**			.25**	.16*
Divorce E	-.03	-.07	-.01	-.30*					
Divorce F	.29*	-.02	-.16	-.01					
Crime P	.27	.06	.02	.32*					.17*
Cancer P	.21	.05	-.33*	.16					
Cancer F	.07	.13	-.03	.34**				.24*	
Death P	.45**	.12	-.04	.20					
Old age E	-.09	-.04	.33*	-.38***				-.21*	.18**
Madness P	.27	.17	-.28*	.13	.22*				
Hunger A	.32*	-.09	.12	-.07			.22*		
Sadness P	.48***	.26	.20	.16	.37***		.34***	.21*	.28***

Note. E = Evaluation, P = Potency, A = Activity.
*p < .05. **p < .01 ***p < .001.

6

cultural variation was plausibly idiosyncratic to the Mexican culture, as is discussed later.

GENERAL DISCUSSION OF THE FINDINGS

In line with Spielberger's (1979) conceptualization of stress and anxiety, the term *threat* was used in this study to describe the subjective perception and interpretation of the 20 critical concepts. The semantic differential appeared to be well suited for evaluating the subjective affective meaning of the concepts that were examined by using this device. Threat was assumed to be reflected in (a) the evaluation of the goodness or badness of a critical concept, (b) the perceived potency of a concept that Osgood, May, and Myron (1975) usually considered as the threatening element of affective meaning, and (c) the activity and degree of familiarity the subject attributed to the critical concept.

There was a large difference between the lower- and middle-class male adolescents in the perceived spread of the threat to be dealt with. If the spread of threat were greater, one might expect that the mean anxiety proneness would be greater in the lower- than in the upper-class male adolescents. Because this was not found to be the case, it would seem that the same quantity was spread differently. However, it may also be that if more situationally specific measures of anxiety proneness were used, greater breadth and amounts of anxiety might be found in lower-class, adolescent Mexican boys.

The subcultural differences found in this study appear to indicate that the sources of threat for lower- and middle-class adolescents are radically different. Of the 13 significant sources of threat for the lower-class adolescents, none were significant in the same direction for the middle class.[2] For the lower-class adolescents, a lower self-evaluation and a more positive (actually less negative) evaluation of pain, separation from school, and insult to the mother were associated with higher anxiety proneness. These findings suggest a dramatic contrast in sources of threat for the two social classes.

In the Mexican culture, to be male carries not only high prestige, but also a correspondingly high responsibility to live up to it. Too much is expected from the men, particularly by women. Moreover, adolescent boys from the lower classes, when compared with those in the higher classes, have fewer resources and opportunities to live up to this idealized role. This may explain the greater anxiety proneness of lower-class adolescents who give a lower evaluation of the self. In attempting to compensate for this negative self-evaluation, the lower-class boy may overcompensate, perhaps unconsciously, and brag that it is not so bad to insult the mother. He may also assert that neither pain nor separation from school are as bad as others say. In both cases, however, he does so at the cost of higher anxiety proneness.[3]

The anxiety proneness of lower-class boys was positively correlated with higher

[2]The lower-class girls coincided only once (power of drunkenness) with the lower-class boys in sources of anxiety. The threatening sources were generally unique to the boys.

[3]For insult to the mother, pain, and evaluation of the self, there were significant mean differences between the lower- and upper-class boys in the interpreted direction, making this compensational bragging interpretation credible. For separation from school, there was no mean difference in evaluation.

perceived potency of sickness, sadness, death, and drunkenness. Given lower-class boys' low self-evaluation and inability to live up to their roles, it seems likely that they would perceive these problems as more threatening than would their upper-middle-class counterparts. In the case of the potency of drunkenness, for which all lower-class students were far more threatened, the real threat posed by a drunken father is more often experienced. This threat, which was valid across all four groups of Mexican adolescents, was acknowledged by a Congressional Commission that noted an alarming use of alcohol in the Mexican society.

For the lower-class boys, the greater their familiarity with insult to the mother and divorce, the greater their anxiety proneness. Self-devaluation in the face of the idealized role seems to explain the higher perceived threat reflected in the higher correlations with activity ratings for sickness and hunger. The more that life was perceived as active by these adolescents (more opportunities for failure?), the greater their anxiety proneness. This may be related to an old tradition in which work, study, and labor in general are considered dangerous and even threatening to health, leading to the "natural" tendency to withdraw through tranquility, immobility, and passiveness (learned helplessness?). It is to be hoped that these attitudes are being overcome, particularly by the Mexican lower classes.

Relatively few of the 20 potentially threatening concepts affected the upper-middle-class boys. The highest correlation of anxiety proneness for this group was with familiarity with separation from school. In contrast to girls, there is greater pressure on boys in the Mexican culture to complete higher education. The affectively perceived potency of pain was the second largest threat for the upper-middle-class boys, and this was also a threat for lower-class boys, but not for the girls of either social class. The Spanish word for pain, *dolor,* means physical pain, but if refers primarily to sentimental pain, which is often pain associated with being in love. In Mexico (witness its songs), romantic love is perceived ambivalently. Although wonderful, romantic love generally involves much suffering, with the man being jilted again and again by the woman. This type of meaning, which has Shakespearean and operatically dramatic elements, may also be partially responsible for the higher positive correlation with evaluation of pain by the lower-class boys.

Not surprisingly, the more negatively sickness was evaluated by the upper-class adolescents, the more anxiety it provoked. In contrast to the girls, the boys in the sample considered the power of sickness, madness, and sadness as highly threatening. The fact that these concepts did not seem to worry the girls apparently reflects the fact that, within the Mexican family, they are much more protected, at least through adolescence.

There were only two sources of anxiety that were common to the girls across social class. The less activity they perceived in themselves and the more activity they perceived in separation from school, the more they were threatened. This was especially true for the upper-class girls. The girls as a group had a higher mean score for activity of the self than did the boys. Although the contrasting interpretation of this source of threat for the boys remains enigmatic, it may be that a lesser possession of this feminine characteristic was threatening.

In a study of the self-concept of Mexicans (Diaz-Guerrero, 1982b), it was found that activity of the self referred fundamentally to communion and expressive activities. It seems likely that a perception of less femininity in themselves was threatening to Mexican adolescent girls. Perceived activity regarding separation from school may have been more threatening to the girls in this study because they were pursuing a high school education and thus differed from most women in Mexico.

For the lower-class girls, greater anxiety proneness was associated with less perceived potency of the self (highest correlation), higher perceived dynamism of insult to the mother, higher potency of drunkenness, higher evaluation of old age, and less potency ascribed to cancer and madness. As was the case for the lower-class boys, a certain exercise of denial appears necessary for the lower-class girls. Thus, the less power they attributed to cancer and madness, the more anxious they were. Vice versa, the more prone they were to anxiety, the less potency they attributed to cancer and madness. Other results were more rational: for example, the greater the threat attributed to drunkenness and insult to the mother, the greater the anxiety proneness.

In striking contrast to the upper-class girls, the less power lower-class girls perceived in themselves, the more anxiety prone they were. These feelings of powerlessness seem to be the Achilles heel for provoking threat in the lower-class girls. The higher the evaluation of old age by the lower-class girls, the more anxiety prone they were, whereas for the middle-class girls, the worse old age was perceived, the higher their trait anxiety. All in all, however, the lower-class girls appeared to be far more protected from various sources of anxiety than their lower-class male counterparts.

In contrast to the lower-class students, the upper-middle-class girls reported more sources of anxiety in responding to the critical concepts than did the upper-class boys. As seen earlier, the less dynamism (femininity?) the girls ascribed to themselves, the more threatened they felt. The more power that upper-class girls attributed to aggression, crime, and separation from school, the more familiar they were with cancer; and the more negatively divorce was evaluated, the more anxious they were. All the these appear to be rational fears.

SUMMARY AND CONCLUSIONS

This exploratory study of cognitions associated with anxiety proneness may raise more questions than it answers. From the two possible causative interpretations, the critical clinical concepts in this study were interpreted as sources of anxiety proneness. Although most of the associations appeared to be rational, there were a few that seemed irrational for which knowledge of the culture permitted a tentative interpretation. Interpretations of the findings in the affective cognition domain explored by the semantic differential technique suggested important psychodynamic defense mechanisms of compensation and denial.

This exploratory study identified specific sources of anxiety in cognition that were subculturally determined. Gender, social class, and their combination appeared to fundamentally influence the type of stimulus situations that were perceived as threatening. A serious approach to clinical psychology must develop blueprints, not only for social class and gender, but for different age levels, in order to better understand the sources of anxiety and the roots of maladjustment and neurosis in a particular society. The results further suggested that universal interpretations, such as the Oedipus complex, as the genesis of human anxiety are somewhat far-fetched, and pointed to the critical importance of the cultural ecosystem in personality development.

REFERENCES

Calatayud, A., Reyes-Lagunes, I., Avila, M. A., & Diaz-Guerrero, R. (1974). *El Perfil de Teleaudiencia de Plaza Sesamo* [Profile of the television audience of Sesamo Plaza]. Mexico City, Mexico: Ediciones INCCAPAC.

Diaz-Guerrero, R. (1979). Origines de la personnalite humaine et des systemes sociaux [Origins of human personality and social systems]. *Revue de Psychologie Appliquée, 29,* 139–152.

Diaz-Guerrero, R. (1980). The culture-counterculture theoretical approach to human and social system development. The case of mothers in four Mexican subcultures. *Proceedings of the Twenty-second International Congress of Psychology* (pp. 55–60). Leipzig, German Democratic Republic.

Diaz-Guerrero, R. (1982a). The psychology of the historic-sociocultural premise, I. *Spanish Language Psychology, 2,* 383–410.

Diaz-Guerrero, R. (1982b). El yo del Mexicano y la Piramide [The self of the Mexican and the pyramid]. In R. Diaz-Guerrero (Ed.), *Psicologia del Mexicano* (pp. 195–241). Mexico City, Mexico: Trillas.

Diaz-Guerrero, R. (1986a). Historio-socio-cultura y personalidad. Definicion y caracteristicas de los factores de la familia mexicana [Social and cultural history and personality. Definition and characteristics of factors in Mexican families]. *Revista de Psicologia Social y Personalidad, 2,* 15–42.

Diaz-Guerrero, R. (1986b). Una etnopsicologia mexicana [A Mexican ethnopsychology]. *Revista de Psicologia Social y Personalidad, 2,* 1–22.

Diaz-Guerrero, R., & Castillo Vales, V. M. (1981). El enfoque cultura-contracultura y el desarrollo cognitivo y de la personalidad en escolares yucatecos [The cultural and countercultural focus and the cognitive and personality development of students in the Yucatan]. *Enseñanza e Investigacion en Psicologia, 7,* 5–26.

Diaz-Guerrero, R., Lichtszajn, J. L., & Reyes Lagunes, I. (1979). Alienacion de la madre, psicopatologia y la practica clinica en Mexico [Alienation from the mother, psychopathology and clinical practice in Mexico]. *Hispanic Journal of Behavioral Sciences, 1,* 117–133.

Diaz-Guerrero, R., & Salas, M. (1975). *El Diferencial Semantico del Idioma Español.* [Semantic differences of the Spanish language]. Mexico City, Mexico: Trillas.

Lichtszajn, J. L. (1979). *Correlatos Clinicos y Socioculturales de la Actitud hacia la Muerte en un Grupo de Adolescentes Mexicanos* [Clinical and sociocultural correlations of the attitudes of a group of Mexican adolescents toward death]. Unpublished doctoral dissertation, Universidad Nacional Autonoma de Mexico, Mexico City, Mexico.

Magnusson, D., Stattin, H., & Iwawaki, S. (1983). Cross-cultural comparisons of situational anxiety reactions. In C. D. Spielberger & R. Diaz-Guerrero (Eds.), *Cross-cultural anxiety* (Vol. 2, pp. 177–190). Washington, DC: Hemisphere.

Osgood, C. E., Suci, G. J., & Tannenbaum, P. H. (1957). *The measurement of meaning.* Urbana: University of Illinois Press.

Osgood, C. E., May, W. H., & Myron, M. S. (1975). Cross-cultural universals of affective meaning. Urbana: University of Illinois Press.

Spielberger. C. D. (1966). *Anxiety and behavior.* New York: Academic Press.

Spielberger, C. D. (1972). *Anxiety: Current trends in theory and research* (Vol. 1). New York: Academic Press.

Spielberger, C. D. (1979). *Understanding stress in anxiety.* New York: Harper & Row.

Spielberger, C. D., & Diaz-Guerrero, R. (1975). IDARE, *Inventario de Ansiedad: Rasgo-Estado* [State-Trait Anxiety Inventory]. Mexico: El Manual Moderno, S.A.

Spielberger, C. D., & Diaz-Guerrero, R. (1976). *Cross-cultural anxiety.* Washington, DC: Hemisphere.

Spielberger, C. D., & Diaz-Guerrero, R. (1983). *Cross-cultural anxiety* (Vol. 2). Washington, DC: Hemisphere.

Spielberger, C. D., & Diaz-Guerrero, R. (1986). *Cross-cultural anxiety* (Vol. 3). Washington, DC: Hemisphere.

Spielberger, C. D., Gorsuch, R. L., & Lushene, R. E. (1970). *State-Trait Anxiety Inventory (Self-evaluation questionnaire).* Palo Alto, CA: Consulting Psychologists Press.

2

Personality Factors in Stress and Anxiety

John Brebner
University of Adelaide, Australia

This chapter is about stress and Eysenck's personality factors of Neuroticism and Introversion–Extraversion, both of which, it is suggested, predispose an individual to being affected by stress and anxiety under conditions that may be present in everyday environments. Neuroticism, or emotional lability, can be related to the experience of stress by the nature of the items on the Neuroticism (N) Scale of the Eysenck Personality Questionnaire, which shows that high scorers are overemotional people, anxious and worrying if introverted, touchy and aggressive if extraverted. Thus, Introversion–Extraversion (E) gives direction to the expression of emotion under stress. This factor has also been linked to the capacity to either be overloaded by strong stimulation or withstand it. Whether high levels of stimulation are stressful in their effects on individuals depends to an important extent on their personalities.

In recent years, psychologists have shown considerable interest in the stress of daily living conditions (Proshansky, Nelson-Shulman, & Kaminoff, 1979). Environmental stressors such as noise (to which many urban inhabitants are inescapably exposed) have been related to a whole range of effects, for example, headaches, tension, fatigue, and sleeping problems (McLean & Tarnopolsky, 1977) or to increased patient-stay periods in hospitals (Fife & Rappaport, 1976). Together with these environmental stressors, some of the interactions with other people that occur in densely populated urban centers seem to affect both skilled performance and social behavior. Among the effects on social behavior, levels of altruism, helping behavior, and honesty are reported to be lower in large cities than in small towns (Korte & Kerr, 1975; Milgram, 1970).

Various forms of skilled performance have been shown to be impaired under very crowded conditions where the conventional distances between people cannot be maintained. One example, which also shows the importance of individual differences (Rawls, Trego, McGaffey, & Rawls, 1972), is a study that found that people who preferred large personal spaces were less successful at arithmetic calculations when made to perform under crowded conditions. However, on the same task, the performance of a group with low personal-space demands actually improved under crowding. Although demonstrating that individual differences are important in reacting to personal-space invasion, this study did not link them to any wider theoretical framework. There are, however, a number of findings that support the view that infringements of personal space produce increased arousal. These allow the suggestion that, theoretically, models of introversion–extraversion may be useful in predicting the effect of personal-space invasion on performance. Whether personal-space invasion is stressful may depend on cultural or contextual factors, but violation of personal space has been singled out as an environmental stressor by previous writers (e.g., Rule & Nesdale, 1976). Siprelle, Ascough, Dietrio, and Horst's (1977) finding that extraverted people became angry under induced affect and introverted people became anxious suggests that both groups were stressed by being crowded.

Findings that support the notion that invasion of personal space creates increased arousal include galvanic skin response (GSR) increasing as an individual is approached by other people (Aiello, DeRisi, Epstein, & Karlin, 1977), heart rate and blood pressure increasing in crowded conditions (Evans, 1975), and palmar sweating increasing under crowding (Saegart, 1974). Differences in how individuals' performances are affected by increased arousal can be predicted from several theories, notably Eysenck's (1967), which suggests that extraversion is associated with low arousal. There is no shortage of empirical support for this view, and the fact that introverted and extraverted people differ in their responsiveness to very low and very high levels of stimulation has been established by many studies. Also, because Gray (1964) set the scene for it, a parallel has often been drawn cautiously between extraversion and strength of the nervous system in Pavlovian terms, at least as far as withstanding intense stimulation and continuing to respond under it (e.g., Fowles, Roberts, & Nagel, 1977).

As far as being stressed is concerned, perhaps the clearest indications that extraverted people do not find intense stimulation as stressing as introverted people comes from studies by Haslam (1972) and Lynn and Eysenck (1961). These studies show that extraverted people have higher thresholds even for pain. At the other end of the intensity scale, various studies have shown that introverted people or those with weak nervous systems have lower sensory thresholds and are more capable of performing tasks that demand continuous attending and that involve searching for weak, infrequent stimuli that are usually unpredictable (Bakan, 1959; Bakan, Belton, & Toth, 1963; Brebner & Cooper, 1974; Eysenck, 1967; Eysenck & Eysenck, 1967; Gray, 1964; Keister & McLaughlin, 1972; Siddle, Morrish, White, & Mangan, 1969; Rozhdestventskaya, Golubeva, & Yermolayeva-Tomina, 1972; Smith, 1968; Strelau, 1970).

What should one expect to happen to the performance of different personality types on difficult and demanding tasks when the tasks are carried out within a reasonably stimulating context? This is an interesting question from a theoretical standpoint. Given the view that extraverted people are typically less aroused than introverted people, extraverts' performances should improve when working under more stimulating conditions, even, as shown in one study (Fraser, 1953), given the presence of just one other person in the room. However, the model of extraversion first put forward by Brebner and Cooper (1974) distinguishes between the central processes concerned with stimulus analysis and response organization and suggests that whether extraverted people's performance is improved depends on the relative demands for these qualities in the task to be carried out and on the task's setting. This model is an attempt to unify the major views of extraversion, most notably Eysenck's reactive inhibition and arousal explanations, into a single theory. To achieve this, Brebner and Cooper's model postulates that introverted people are characterized by a tendency to derive excitation from stimulus analysis but inhibition from response organization. Extraverted people have the opposite tendency, generating excitation from response organization and inhibition from stimulus analysis.

Excitation can be defined as the tendency to continue or to augment a particular form of behavior; *inhibition,* as the tendency to discontinue or attenuate it. The central process of response organization precedes the actual emitting of responses that themselves generate further stimuli for analysis. The analysis of these response-mediated stimuli has an inhibitory effect in extraverted individuals, so that, through continued responding, extraverts tend to build up an inhibitory state, whereas introverted individuals do not. This is rather like the original reactive inhibition theory offered by Eysenck (1957). The unified model tends to make the same predictions as that theory and the later one in terms of arousal levels.

Under increased stimulation produced by invasion of personal space, however, the model predicts that, rather than improving because of higher arousal, extraverted people's performance should be *adversely* affected at tasks that are high in demands for stimulus analysis and therefore produce an inhibitory state in extraverts. This prediction was tested by Katsikitis and Brebner (1981), using two versions of a letter-cancellation task. One task involved crossing out every letter *a* and demanded less in the way of stimulus analysis than the other task, which required four letters, *w, m, n,* and *c,* to be cancelled. The number of letters that should have been cancelled but were missed was used as the measure of performance.

The main finding was that the three-way interaction, Extraversion × Being Crowded × Task Difficulty, was significant. As predicted, the performance of the extraverted subjects suffered when they were faced with a difficult task under crowded conditions (see Table 1). The N factor also seemed to be relevant, with high scorers missing significantly more signals than did low scorers (on average, 69.5 compared with 47.6). However, the most relevant interaction, Neuroticism × Extraversion × Being Crowded × Task Difficulty, approached significance, $F(1, 56) = 3.84$, but did not reach the 0.05 level = 4.02.

These results were obtained under interpersonal-spacing conditions. In the crowded condition, 8 subjects were seated in a 2.68 m × 1.26 m room on chairs only 0.1 m apart, which is a smaller space than in some other studies (e.g., Meisels & Canter, 1970). The small space ensured that subjects rubbed shoulders with their neighbors and touched knees with the person opposite them. Although such conditions are likely to raise arousal levels, no physiological data were recorded in this study.

A questionnaire administered to the 64 subjects immediately after the experiment indicated that introverted subjects did tend to be more anxious than their extraverted counterparts. In terms of the group's performance being stressed by

Table 1 Mean Number of Missed Letters

	Level of crowding	
Level of task	Noncrowded	Crowded
Easy		
Introverts	43.3	54.6
Extraverts	34.1	42.6
Difficult		
Introverts	67.5	70.3
Extraverts	60.6	95.4

the invasion of personal space, however, it was clearly the extraverted subjects who failed to cope with the difficult task when crowded. This was expected because the task and its setting were high in demands for stimulus analysis. The same result would not be predicted for tasks with greater requirements for response organization because these tasks would tend to produce excitation in extraverts, which would maintain their level of performance. In tasks where demands for response organization predominate, the model predicts that introverted individuals' responsiveness would be lowered because, for them, response organization would generate inhibition.

Relative to extraverted individuals, introverted individuals' predisposition to derive inhibition from response organization reduces the likelihood of their responding. This, in some circumstances, makes them more ready to learn not to respond. This aspect of the model can be linked to "learned helplessness" (Seligman, 1975) and gives rise to the prediction that there will be differences between introverted and extraverted individuals in whether they tend to become "helpless" or not. *Learned helplessness* refers to a deficit in performance that results from exposure to events that the individual cannot control. This effect has been shown in human and animal subjects and was originally explained in terms of the individual's learning that there is no relation between their responses and events that occur. If an individual expects events in the environment to be independent of their responses and, therefore, outside of their control, their capacity to interact effectively with their environment is impaired.

A reformulation of the learned helplessness theory (Abramson, Seligman, & Teasdale, 1978) includes the causes to which the individual attributes his or her lack of control over events. However, whatever attributions are made, people who learn to become helpless are less able to make appropriate responses to reduce the effects of external stressors, and their perceived lack of control can itself be a lasting source of stress. Indeed, learning that responses and outcomes are independent of each other has been suggested to underlie states of reactive depression (Seligman, Klein, & Miller, 1976). Individual differences in susceptibility to learned helplessness have been suggested previously. Stokols (1979), for example, reported that people with an external rather than an internal locus of control are more prone to develop learned helplessness following exposure to uncontrollable aversive events.

Typically, studies of learned helplessness proceed in two stages. First, subjects undergo a training session in which they attempt to gain control over some effect, for example, trying to turn off a loud, high-pitched noise. The training task is either controllable (i.e., it is possible to learn to control the effect) or uncontrollable (i.e., nothing the subject does has the desired effect). A controllable test task follows the training session. Subjects who undergo uncontrollable training show more helplessness in the test task. Helplessness is usually evidenced by how often the subject fails to control the effect, by the average time taken to make responses, and the number of trials to some criterion (e.g., three successive, successful responses). The conditional probability of a failure to control, given a successful attempt to control on the previous trial, is also used as a measure of helplessness.

The circumstances in which the new model of extraversion predicts that introverted individuals will become helpless after an uncontrollable training task require the training and test tasks to be high on response organization but low on stimulus-analysis demands. In controllable training, success leads all subjects to respond selectively and in the same way. During uncontrollable training, although all subjects are unsuccessful, the organization of responses in the attempt to control will create an excitatory tendency in extraverted subjects but an inhibitory one in introverted subjects. This will carry over into the test phase and, by lowering the responsiveness of introverted subjects during that phase, will favor the production of learned helplessness in those subjects.

This prediction was tested (Tiggemann, Winefield, & Brebner, 1982) by using a quiet, nonaversive buzzer that subjects attempted to switch off. In the controllable test phase, subjects had two response buttons. Any combination that included pressing the left button once and the right button twice terminated the buzzer. Because in the test phase the lowest probability of success for any sequence of only three responses was 0.375, it is unlikely that any failure to control the buzzer reflected an inability to find correct controlling responses. Rather, helplessness, if it is induced by uncontrollable training, will be likely to be mediated by lowered responsiveness and is more likely to be found in introverted subjects.

Forty-eight student subjects took part in this experiment. Half of them were introverts with an average score of 6.2 on the E Scale of the EPQ; the others were extraverts with an average score of 18.3 on the E Scale. Table 2 summarizes the results and shows that, as predicted, after uncontrollable training the introverted subjects exhibited significantly higher levels of helplessness on all four of the measures used. Following controllable training, only one measure, number of failures, showed a significant difference between groups, and here it was the extraverted subjects who failed more often. Although Neuroticism was also controlled, it was not a significant effect and did not interact with any other variable. This lack of a neuroticism effect was predicted on the grounds that, unlike helplessness experiments that use aversive stimuli, the present arrangements would not produce emotional reactions in subjects.

These two experiments offer further support for the view that extraverted and introverted people generate inhibition from stimulus analysis and response organization, respectively. The fact that, in the first experiment, extraverted subjects only missed more signals than introverted subjects when performing the difficult task under crowding shows that impairment acts specifically on their capacity to analyze stimuli. This particular finding has been replicated in a more recent experiment by Khew and Brebner (1985), and other studies have also tested predictions from the model successfully, in several cases using reaction-time methods (see Brebner, 1980, 1983). The two experiments presented here, however, chose personal space invasion and exposure to uncontrollable effects to test the model's relevance for two of the stresssors identified in environmental psychology as occurring quite generally in urban environments.

It is of some interest that although introverted subjects are more easily over-

Table 2 Mean Values for Four Measures of Learned Helplessness for Introverts (I) and Extraverts (E)

Training	Response latency		Number of failures		Trials to criterion		Conditional probability	
	I	E	I	E	I	E	I	E
Controllable	6.40	5.90	0.25	0.90	3.42	3.59	.010	.018
Uncontrollable	8.17	6.93	8.25	3.34	11.25	6.33	.34	.11

loaded by strong stimulation, these subjects were able to maintain their level of performance on the highly "inspective" letter-cancellation task under crowding even though they tended to report experiencing more anxiety than did extraverted subjects. This is in line with previous results. For example, Schalling (1975) showed that measures that included muscle tension and anticipatory worrying correlated positively with neuroticism but negatively with extraversion. Eysenck (1975) has pointed out the importance of introversion–extraversion in conjunction with neuroticism for the formation of neurotic disorders and anxiety reactions under stressful conditions. High neuroticism together with introversion predisposes the individual to produce relatively strong fear reactions that are easily conditioned, and trait anxiety, as measured by the Manifest Anxiety Scale, is positively related to introversion and neuroticism (Eysenck & Eysenck, 1969).

After the helplessness experiment, introverted subjects rated themselves on a 6-point scale as being less satisfied with their performance on the uncontrollable training task than did extraverts. However, rather than being induced by the tasks alone, these reports could reflect a more generalized tendency for introverted subjects to have a more negative view of themselves and the things that happen to them. Various findings lend themselves to this suggestion (e.g., Fremont, Means, & Means, 1970; Kawash, 1982; Verma & Upadhay, 1980). It is easy to argue that people whose characteristics include finding it stressful to have to deal with strong stimulation, needing to integrate information over relatively long periods before reaching decisions, and being prone to effects like learned helplessness will, by generalization, develop a negative view of their own ability to interact successfully with their environment and with other people.

Evidence for this was found in responses to a questionnaire we are developing that measures the degree of satisfaction people express about a range of different holiday experiences. When answering questions about how satisfied they are with various activities, or how enjoyable they find them, the respondents' status as introverted or extraverted, as well as their neuroticism, is again very relevant to their responses. Table 3 gives the means for each of eight items for five groups of students with different scores on E and N. The responses are expressed as percentages, so that, in this set of items, the higher the mean, the greater the expressed satisfaction or enjoyment. These data were obtained from students in their first week at the university, when they were undergoing many of the same, or similar, experiences.

It is clear from Table 3 that extraverted subjects with low neuroticism responded most favorably and introverted subjects high on neuroticism responded least favorably. However, extraverted subjects with high neuroticism scores and ambiverted subjects with moderate neuroticism scores are quite similar, and both give more favorable responses than either of the introverted groups, even those introverted subjects with moderate scores on neuroticism.

CONCLUSIONS AND SUMMARY

In summary, these studies taken together show three things. First, they point to the importance of introversion–extraversion, as well as neuroticism, in assessing the effect of environmental stressors. Second, beyond that, the first two experiments support the general prescription from the new model of extraversion that,

Table 3 Mean Response Values for Five Groups of Subjects with Different Extraversion (*E*) and Neuroticism (*N*) Scores

	LEHN ($n = 32$)	LEMN ($n = 31$)	MEMN ($n = 44$)	HEHN ($n = 27$)	HELN ($n = 46$)
What percent of your time in the past few days has been spent in places that could be called beautiful or attractive?					
M	42.2	39.7	50.7	49.6	56.5
SD	24.19	24.96	26.62	25.19	26.93
What percent of your time during the past few days have you actually spent enjoying yourself?					
M	44.4	49.4	64.8	63.3	65.0
SD	29.83	23.51	26.72	22.53	23.36
What percent of the past few days was spent in leisure or recreational activities which you liked doing?					
M	35.6	39.0	48.4	53.3	52.2
SD	26.87	23.29	26.14	25.27	26.74
How much of tomorrow do you expect to be enjoyable?					
M	53.8	65.5	71.1	71.5	78.3
SD	23.79	20.63	17.94	18.12	20.03
How much have you enjoyed the scenery you have seen today?					
M	44.4	52.3	51.8	52.6	61.1
SD	30.26	26.80	28.55	29.95	28.30
What percent of the food you have eaten in the past few days would you rate as delicious?					
M	41.3	52.3	59.8	57.8	64.6
SD	26.49	24.73	27.99	26.65	28.57
How enjoyable have you found any tourist visits or trips you have taken in the last few days?					
M	37.8	49.0	56.4	55.9	66.1
SD	35.26	31.24	33.35	33.66	32.90
To what degree have your hopes and expectations of what things would be like been satisfied over the past few days?					
M	50.6	54.2	58.6	57.0	61.1
SD	27.93	23.63	25.30	26.86	24.61

Note. Low (L) = +0.5 *SD* below mean, moderate (M) = within 0.5 *SD* of mean, high (H) = +0.5 *SD* above mean.

other things being equal, introverted and extraverted subjects will find more difficulty in overcoming their inherent inhibitory tendencies under task demands for response organization and stimulus analysis, respectively. Third, in supporting the new model, these studies show that we can now identify, with a reasonable degree of precision, some of the mechanisms that mediate the effects of the stress-producing situations people meet in their everyday urban environments.

REFERENCES

Abramson, L. Y., Seligman, M. E. P., & Teasdale, J. D. (1978). Learned helplessness in humans: Critique and reformulation. *Journal of Abnormal Psychology, 87,* 49–74.

Aiello, J. R., DeRisi, D. T., Epstein, Y. M., & Karlin, R. A. (1977). Crowding and the role of interpersonal distance preference. *Sociometry, 40,* 271–282.

Bakan, P. (1959). Extraversion-introversion and improvement in an auditory vigilance task. *British Journal of Psychology, 50,* 325–332.

Bakan, P., Belton, J., & Toth, J. (1963). Extraversion-introversion and decrement in an auditory vigilance task. In D. N. Buckner & J. J. McGrath (Eds.), *Vigilance: A symposium* (pp. 22–33). New York: McGraw-Hill.

Brebner, J. (1980). Reaction time in personality theory. In A. T. Welford (Ed.), *Reaction times.* London: Academic Press.

Brebner, J. (1983). A model of extraversion. *Australian Journal of Psychology, 35,* 349–359.

Brebner, J., & Cooper, C. (1974). The effect of a low rate of regular signals upon the reaction times of introverts and extraverts. *Journal of Research in Personality, 8,* 263–276.

Evans, G. W. (1975). *Behavioural and physiological consequences of crowding in humans.* Unpublished doctoral thesis, University of Massachusetts, Amherst.

Eysenck, H. J. (1957). *The dynamics of anxiety and hysteria.* London: Routledge & Kegan Paul.

Eysenck, H. J. (1967). *The biological basis of personality.* Springfield, IL: Charles C Thomas.

Eysenck, H. J. (1975). A genetic model of anxiety. In I. G. Sarason & C. D. Spielberger (Eds.), *Stress and anxiety* (Vol. 2, pp. 81–116). Washington, DC: Hemisphere.

Eysenck, H. J., & Eysenck, S. B. G. (1967). Physiological reactivity to sensory stimulation as a measure of personality. *Psychological Reports, 20,* 45–46.

Eysenck, H. J., & Eysenck, S. B. G. (1969). *Personality structure and measurement.* London: Routledge & Kegan Paul.

Fife, D., & Rappaport, E. (1976). Noise and hospital stay. *American Journal of Public Health, 66,* 680–681.

Fowles, D. C., Roberts, R., & Nagel, K. E. (1977). The influence of introversion/extraversion on the skin conductance response to stress and stimulus intensity. *Journal of Research in Personality, 11,* 129–146.

Fraser, D. C. (1953). The relation of an environmental variable to performance in a prolonged visual task. *Quarterly Journal of Experimental Psychology, 5,* 31–32.

Fremont, T., Means, G. H., & Means, R. S. (1970). Anxiety as a function of task performance feedback and extraversion-introversion. *Psychological Reports, 27,* 455–458.

Gray, J. A. (Ed.). (1964). *Pavlov's typology.* Oxford: Pergamon Press.

Haslam, D. R. (1972). Experimental pain. In V. D. Nebylitsyn & J. A. Gray (Eds.), *Biological bases of individual differences* (pp. 242–253). London: Academic Press.

Katsikitis, M., & Brebner, J. (1981). Individual differences in the effects of personal space invasion: A test of the Brebner-Cooper model of extraversion. *Personality and Individual Differences, 2,* 5–10.

Kawash, G. F. (1982). A structural analysis of self-esteem from pre-adolescence through young adulthood: Anxiety and extraversion as agents in the development of self-esteem. *Journal of Clinical Psychology, 38,* 301–311.

Keister, M. E., & McLaughlin, R. J. (1972). Vigilance performance related to extraversion-introversion and caffeine. *Journal of Research in Personality, 6,* 5–11.

Khew, K., & Brebner, J. (1985). The role of personality in crowding research. *Personality and Individual Differences, 6,* 641–643.

Korte, C., & Kerr, N. (1975). Responses to altruistic opportunities under urban and rural conditions. *Journal of Social Psychology, 95,* 183–184.

Lynn, R., & Eysenck, H. J. (1961). Tolerance for pain, extraversion and neuroticism. *Perceptual and Motor Skills, 12,* 161–162.

McLean, E. K., & Tarnopolsky, A. (1977). Noise discomfort and mental health. A review of the socio-medical implications of disturbance by noise. *Psychological Medicine, 7,* 19–62.

Meisels, M., & Canter, F. M. (1970). Personal space and personality characteristics: A non-confirmation. *Psychological Reports, 27,* 287–290.

Milgram, S. (1970). The experience of living in cities. *Science, 167,* 1461–1468.

Proshansky, H. M., Nelson-Shulman, Y., & Kaminoff, D. (1979). The role of physical settings in life-crisis experience. In I. G. Sarason & C. D. Spielberger (Eds.), *Stress and anxiety* (Vol. 6, pp. 3–25). Washington, DC: Hemisphere.

Rawls, J. R., Trego, R. E., McGaffey, C. N., & Rawls, D. J. (1972). Personal space as a predictor of performance under close working conditions. *Journal of Social Psychology, 86,* 261-267.

Rozhdestventskaya, V. L., Golubeva, E. A., & Yermolayeva-Tomina, L. B. (1972). Alterations in functional state as affected by different kinds of activity and strength of the nervous system. In V. D. Nebylitsin & J. A. Gray (Eds.), *Biological bases of individual behavior* (pp. 291-309). London: Academic Press.

Rule, B. G., & Nesdale, A. R. (1976). Environmental stressors, emotional arousal, and aggression. In I. G. Sarason & C. D. Spielberger (Eds.), *Stress and anxiety* (Vol. 3, pp. 87-103.). Washington, DC: Hemisphere.

Saegart, S. (1974). *Effects of spatial and social density on arousal, mood and social orientation.* Unpublished doctoral thesis, University of Michigan.

Schalling, D. S. (1975). Types of anxiety and types of stressors as related to personality. In I. G. Sarason & C. D. Spielberger (Eds.), *Stress and anxiety* (Vol. 3, pp. 49-71). Washington, DC: Hemisphere.

Seligman, M. E. P. (1975). *Helplessness.* San Francisco: Freeman.

Seligman, M. E. P., Klein, D. C., & Miller, W. R. (1976). Depression. In H. Leitenberg (Ed.), *Handbook of behaviour modification.* Englewood Cliffs, NJ: Prentice-Hall.

Siddle, D. A. T., Morrish, R. B., White, K. D., & Mangan, G. L. (1969). Relation of visual sensitivity to extraversion. *Journal of Research in Personality, 3,* 264-267.

Siprelle, R. E., Ascough, J. C., Dietrio, D. M., & Horst, P. A. (1977). Neuroticism, extroversion and response to stress. *Behaviour Research and Therapy, 15,* 411-418.

Smith, S. L. (1968). Extraversion and sensory threshold. *Psychophysiology, 5,* 293-299.

Stokols, D. (1979). A congruence analysis of human stress. In I. G. Sarason & C. D. Spielberger (Eds.), *Stress and anxiety* (Vol. 6, pp. 27-53). Washington, DC: Hemisphere.

Strelau, J. (1970). Nervous system type and extraversion-introversion: A comparison of Eysenck's theory with Pavlov's typology. *Polish Psychological Bulletin, 1,* 17-24.

Tiggemann, M., Winefield, A. H., & Brebner, J. (1982). The role of extraversion in the development of learned helplessness. *Personality and Individual Differences, 3,* 27-34.

Verma, O. P., & Upadhay, S. N. (1980). Extraversion in relation to conflict and anxiety. *Indian Psychological Review, 19,* 16-19.

3

Emotional Patterns in Stress Situations and Somatic Diseases

Kazimierz Wrzesniewski
Warsaw Medical Academy, Poland

Evidence that psychological factors play an important role in the onset and development of somatic diseases has accumulated for more than half a century. This evidence comes from five different research approaches. The first consists of animal experiments in the tradition of Cannon, Pavlov, Selye, and Brady, which have shown that significant vegetative changes occur in animals exposed to stressful situations. Similarly, the results of studies of the human subjects' reactions in laboratory and natural stress conditions have shown that humans, like animals, undergo significant physiological changes in stressful situations.

A third group of studies has investigated differences in the personality and life history of healthy people and patients afflicted with various somatic disorders. Although no unequivocal personality profiles have been found to be characteristic of people with particular diseases, certain personality traits seem to differentiate persons with disease from healthy individuals. It has also been reported that, in the life histories of patients suffering from chronic disorders, many more negative situations have occurred than in the life histories of persons in good health. Such findings have been confirmed in methodologically sound prospective studies.

In a fourth group of studies in which demographic variables were investigated, certain somatic diseases were found to occur more often in highly industrialized countries than in developing countries, and in large urban centers as compared with small localities and rural areas. The results of a fifth group of sociological investigations have demonstrated that persons in certain professions are more often afflicted with particular somatic diseases than individuals employed in other, less-stressful occupations.

In all five areas of research, clarifying the role of emotion in the etiology of somatic disorders emerged as a significant issue. Emotions appear to be directly linked to the onset of pathophysiological changes by vegetative-somatic processes, which constitute a major component of emotion. The fact that the frequent experience of negative emotions in stressful situations may accelerate the onset of somatic disorders raises two fundamental questions. Why do some persons exposed to stressful situations become ill and others confronted with the same conditions remain healthy? Why do similar stressors produce a particular disorder (e.g., stomach ulcers) in some people, and others develop a different disorder (e.g., coronary heart disease)?

These questions are partially answered by theories of somatic disease, which postulate that the effects of stress on the onset of a given disorder are mediated by extrapsychological factors, such as genetic endowment, feeding habits, cigarette smoking, and so forth. Such answers are not satisfactory for most psychologists, however, because of strong evidence that people differ in their emotional reactions to stressful situations (Aragon, 1970; Beck, 1972; Borkovec, 1976; Cameron, 1944; Lacey, Bateman, & Van Lehn, 1953; Lacey & Lacey, 1958; Steptoe, 1980). Moreover, the emotional reaction patterns that are characteristic of an individual seem to be relatively independent of the nature of the stressor situation.

The main hypothesis examined in the research reported in this chapter is that individuals afflicted with a particular somatic disease experience different emotional reactions under stressful conditions than do persons who develop a different disease. A corollary is that patients with a particular disease differ from healthy persons in their emotional reactions to stressful situations. More specifically, it is predicted that patients with different somatic disorders tested in the same situation will differ from each other in their emotional reactions to stress, and that the emotional reactions of sick individuals will differ from those of an equivalent group of healthy persons. Verification of these hypotheses was undertaken by P. Lepczynski (1983) as part of his master's thesis.

METHOD

Subjects

Three groups of 20 male subjects, matched for age, education, and occupation, participated in the study. All subjects were white-collar employees, aged 35–55, with college or other academic education. The first group consisted of myocardial infarction (MI) patients, with no complications and no other diseases, who were undergoing posthospital rehabilitation in a sanatorium. The second group consisted of peptic ulcer (PU) patients, with no other disease, undergoing sanatorium treatment. Employees of an office in Warsaw constituted the third group; medical examinations found the subjects in this group to be free of any affliction.

Measures

Two major components of the subjects' emotional reactions to stress were evaluated: the content and intensity of emotional experience and physiological changes. A Polish adaptation (Wrzesniewski, 1984) of Spielberger's (1979) State–Trait Personality Inventory (STPI) was used to assess emotional experience. The theoretical principles that guided the construction of the STPI, which consists of six subscales for measuring state and trait anxiety, curiosity, and anger, were the same as those that guided the development of Spielberger's well-known anxiety scales (Spielberger, Gorsuch, & Lushene, 1970). Three important characteristics of the STPI make this inventory especially useful for assessing subjective emotional experience: (a) The STPI permits differentiation between anxiety and anger, the two emotions that are most common in stress situations; (b) it is brief and easy to administer and score; and (c) it can be administered repeatedly over short intervals.

The physiological manifestations of emotion that were measured in this study were systolic and diastolic blood pressure (SBP and DBP, respectively) and heart rate (HR). These measures were selected because one of the experimental groups consisted of MI patients, for whom cardiovascular reactivity was expected to be a significant factor. The measurement of HR and blood pressure (BP) is also relatively simple and easily managed in laboratory research.

Procedures

Each subject was tested individually under the same laboratory conditions. A stressful situation was created by giving the Raven's test, with a 10-min time limit. The subjects were informed that they were taking an intelligence test and that they should be able to complete it without error within the specified time limit. A stop watch was prominently activated by the experimenter when the subject began. Additional stress was introduced by informing the subject how much time was left and by expressing doubt about whether he would be able to complete the task.

The STPI emotional state measures were administered on three occasions: (a) in a neutral situation shortly after the initial contact with the subject, (b) immediately following the stress situation, and (c) at the conclusion of the experiment, 25 min after the stress situation. The STPI trait scales were given only once, at the time the first STPI state measures were taken. Between the second and third measures, the experimenter engaged the subjects in a neutral conversation about films they had seen, hobbies, and so forth.

Physiological measures were obtained on eight different occasions. The first set of measures was taken shortly after initial contact and before the subject responded to the STPI. The second set of measures was taken in the stress situation, 5 min after the subjects began working on the Raven's test; they were informed that the time required to take BP and HR would be excluded from the 10-min time limit. The third set of measures was taken immediately after the completion of the stressor task. During the neutral conversation, four sets of physiological measures were taken at five-min intervals. The final (eighth) set of physiological measures was taken after the completion of the experiment.

RESULTS

Differences in the Pattern of Emotional Reactions

The mean STPI scores for MI patients, PU patients, and the healthy control group in the initial situation are reported in Table 1. Only one significant difference in the personality traits was found: MI patients scored significantly higher than the healthy controls in trait curiosity. The state anxiety (S-Anxiety) and state anger (S-Anger) scores of the MI patients were lower than those of the other groups, differing significantly from the healthy persons in S-Anxiety and from the PU patients in S-Anger. There are two plausible interpretations of these data: (a) The lower anxiety and anger scores of the MI patients may have resulted from the effects of drugs such as beta-blockers, or (b) these patients may have been using a strong denial mechanism to prevent themselves from experiencing their negative emotions. The findings to be reported for the physiological measures will facilitate discrimination between these interpretations.

Table 1 Means and Standard Deviations for State and Trait Anxiety, Anger, and Curiosity of Myocardial Infarction (MI) and Peptic Ulcer (PU) Patients and Healthy Controls in the Initial Neutral Situation

	Emotional states			Personality traits		
Groups	Anxiety	Anger	Curiosity	Anxiety	Anger	Curiosity
MI patients						
M	16.80	11.80	29.25	21.50	19.00	30.55
SD	4.47	2.69	3.57	2.95	3.88	3.76
PU patients						
M	19.25	14.15	28.65	23.40	21.35	28.70
SD	4.79	4.28	3.39	4.45	5.37	4.09
Healthy controls						
M	20.45	13.95	28.25	21.25	18.50	27.80
SD	5.05	4.69	3.71	3.37	6.12	3.97

The subjective emotional states of the MI and PU patients and the healthy control group in the initial situation, the stress situation, and 25 min later are presented in Table 2, in which it can be noted that the state curiosity (S-Curiosity) scores for all three groups were stable across the three measurement periods. The S-Anxiety and S-Anger scores of the MI patients were higher in the stress situation than in the initial and final situations, but only the S-Anxiety difference was statistically significant. Although the pattern of change in the emotional states of the PU patients was similar to that of the MI patients, the S-Anxiety and S-Anger scores for these patients were markedly and significantly higher during the stress period than during the final period.

Table 2 Means and Standard Deviations for State Anxiety, State Anger and State Curiosity for Myocardial Infarction (MI) and Peptic Ulcer (PU) Patients and Healthy Controls in Three Situations

	State anxiety			State anger			State curiosity		
Groups	1	2	3	1	2	3	1	2	3
MI patients									
M	16.80	19.85	16.15	11.80	12.30	10.95	29.25	29.65	29.45
SD	4.47	2.98	3.25	2.69	3.76	2.72	3.57	4.84	4.36
	x– – – –x x———x								
PU patients									
M	19.25	21.60	16.95	14.15	15.25	12.30	28.65	28.95	29.25
SD	4.79	4.20	4.27	4.28	4.39	3.21	3.39	3.35	3.38
	x———x			x– – – –x					
Healthy controls									
M	20.45	19.80	17.10	13.95	13.20	11.55	28.25	29.05	29.50
SD	5.05	3.97	4.19	4.69	3.94	3.31	3.71	4.02	3.27
	x– – – – – – – – – –x								
	x– – – – –x								

Note. 1 = initial situation, 2 = stress situation, 3 = 25 min later.
x– – – – – –x $p < .05$
x———x $p < .01$

The pattern of S-Anxiety and S-Anger scores for the healthy group differed substantially from that of the two patient groups, as can be seen in Table 2. The anxiety and anger levels were highest for the healthy group in the initial "neutral" situation, decreased slightly in the stress situation, and were significantly lower 25 min later—following the neutral conversation—than in either the initial or the stress situation. These results were quite puzzling, especially the higher anger and anxiety scores in the initial "neutral" situation. The finding that the initial S-Anxiety of the healthy subjects was higher than that of the two patient groups may be related to the fact that these subjects were tested in their job setting. Although they could have refused to participate and were assured that their responses would be used only for scientific purposes, they might still have feared that their job performance was being evaluated and that refusal would put them at a disadvantage. The decrease in anxiety during the experiment corresponds with other studies in which anxiety levels in anticipation of threat were higher than in the real situation (Sosnowski & Wrzesniewski, 1983).

To summarize the results (a) as far as the personality traits are concerned, the MI patients were significantly higher in trait curiosity (T-Curiosity) than the other two groups, but no significant differences among the groups were found in trait anxiety and trait anger (T-Anxiety and T-Anger, respectively); (b) the dynamics of anxiety and anger in both patients' groups differed from those of the healthy persons; (c) although the pattern of change in the emotional states for the two patient groups were similar, only the rise and fall in S-Anxiety for the MI patient and the decline in S-Anxiety and S-Anger from the stress to the final period for the PU patients were statistically significant; and (d) no differences were found in S-Curiosity.

Differences in the Pattern of Physiological Changes

Physiological assessments were taken eight times during the experiment: after contact had been established, in the middle and at the end of the stress situation, and at 5-min intervals during the 25-min neutral conversation period. Mean SBPS for the MI and PU patients and the healthy control group are presented in Figure 1 for the eight measurement periods. The SBP dynamics of healthy persons differed from those of the sick, and the two patient groups also differed from each other. The multivariate analysis of variance indicated statistically significant differences in SBP between the groups as well as differences within each group.

Among the MI patients, SBP was lowest in the initial period, rose steeply during the stress situation, reaching its highest level, and then decreased slowly. Even 25 min after the conclusion of Raven's test, SBP was still slightly higher for the MI patients than it had been in the initial period. The changes in the SBP of the PU patients were quite different from those of the MI patients. For the PU patients, SBP was highest in the initial situation, decreased to its lowest point by the end of the stress situation, and then gradually increased during the 25-min neutral conversation period. For the healthy controls, SBP increased from the first to the second assessment and then decreased, returning to normal 5 min after the conclusion of the stress situation and remaining at this level until the end of the experiment.

The mean DBPS for the three groups are reported in Figure 2. Changes in DBP mirrored those observed for SBP, but were smaller in magnitude. The between-groups differences for DBP were statistically significant, and the statistical findings for both the direction and the time of change were similar to those found for SBP.

The mean HRS for the three experimental groups are presented in Figure 3. The HR changes for the MI and PU patients were similar to those found for blood pressure: HR increased in the MI group and decreased in the PU group during the stress situation, and the direction of change was reversed during the 25-min conversation period. However, the between-groups differences diminished 5 min after the end of the stress situation, and these differences were no longer statistically significant. Although the HR changes in the healthy control group were similar to those in the MI patients, the magnitude of the increase during the stress situation was slight and not statistically significant, and HR returned to the initial level by the end of the stress situation.

Summing up the findings for the dynamics of the physiological measures, the three groups clearly showed different patterns of change. In response to stress, SBP, DBP, and HR increased in the MI patients and decreased in the PU patients. Clearly, the patient groups differed markedly from one another in their cardiovascular reactions to stress, and both patient groups differed from the healthy control group in variability, as in the time required to return to initial levels following stress.

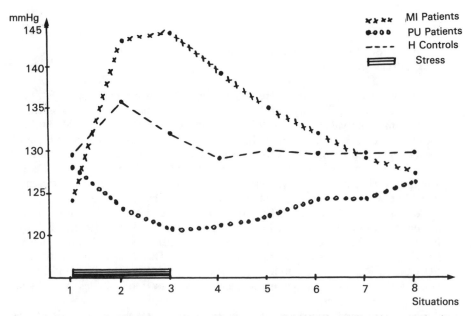

Figure 1 Mean systolic blood pressure in mm/Hg for myocardial infarction (MI) patients, peptic ulcer (PU) patients, and the healthy (H) control group taken before, during, and immediately after performing on a stressful task, and at 5-min intervals during a 25-min neutral conversation.

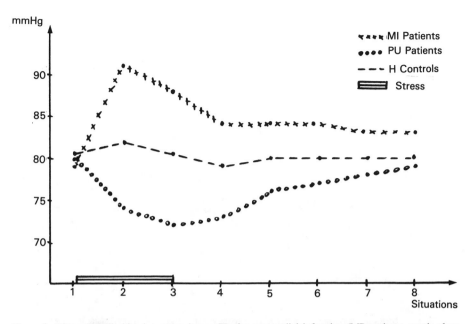

Figure 2   Mean diastolic blood pressure in mm/Hg for myocardial infarction (MI) patients, peptic ulcer (PU) patients, and the healthy (H) control group taken before, during, and immediately after performing on a stressful task, and at 5-min intervals during a 25-min neutral conversation.

DISCUSSION

Before considering the results of this study in the context of related findings reported by other investigators, I would like to comment on the concept of denial as a mechanism for modifying the pattern of emotional reaction. Hackett and Cassem (1974) treated denial as a defense mechanism, which involves "the conscious or unconscious repudiation of part or all of the total available meaning of an event to allay fear, anxiety or other unpleasant affects" (p. 94). Derived from psychoanalysis, this definition differentiates between denial and the well-known defense mechanisms of repression and suppression in terms of distortion of the meaning of an event that evokes anxiety.

In reporting the STPI findings, I suggested that the low S-Anxiety and S-Anger scores of the MI patients might have resulted either from denial or from taking certain drugs such as beta-blockers. If the low emotional state scores resulted from the action of beta-blockers, only small changes in the physiological measures would be expected in the stress situation because these drugs reduce the mobility of vegetative processes. Figures 1, 2, and 3 clearly show that the stress situation produced a sharp increase in all three physiological indicators for the MI patients.

Additional evidence that the MI patients in the present study used denial comes from results obtained with a questionnaire that was given immediately after the stress situation in order to assess subjective awareness of vegetative-somatic changes (Mandler, Mandler, & Uviller, 1958). The finding that the MI patients had

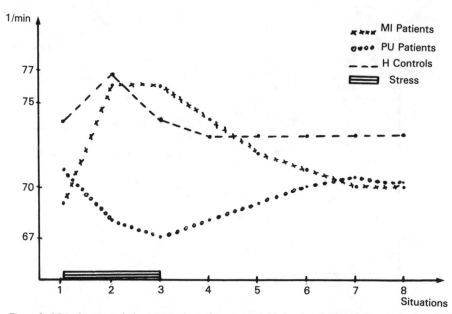

Figure 3 Mean heart rate in beats per minute for myocardial infarction (MI) patients, peptic ulcer (PU) patients, and the healthy (H) control group taken before, during, and immediately after performing on a stressful task, and at 5-min intervals during a 25-min neutral conversation.

the lowest scores on this questionnaire suggested that denial contributed to the low S-Anxiety and S-Anger scores of the MI patients in the initial situation.

The importance of psychodynamic mechanisms of denial, repression, and suppression was emphasized in classical psychosomatic research, but most of the early studies were based primarily on clinical observation and intuition rather than on empirical research. However, in recent studies, many of the early suppositions have been confirmed in scientific investigations (see, among others, Croog & Levine, 1977; Hackett & Cassem, 1974; Lazowski, 1978; Pleszewski, 1977; Reykowski & Krawczyk, 1972). The findings in the present study suggested that the destructive impact of denial may have resulted from the persistence of vegetative changes that differentiated the two patient groups from the healthy control group after the cessation of the stressful situation.

A similar relation was found in a study of matched pairs of men, one of whom was an MI patient and the other of whom had no somatic complaints (Wrzesniewski, 1980). On the basis of information about the emotional reactions to typical, real-life frustrations obtained in standard, structured interviews, the MI patients were found to use the denial mechanism more often, and to experience longer-lasting negative emotions than the group with no somatic complaints. The tendency for vegetative reactions to persist in MI patients was also found by Valek and Kühn (1970), who compared stress-induced changes in MI patients and an equivalent group of healthy persons. Reykowski and Krawczyk (1972) have reported similar relations for gastrological patients for whom the persistence of vegetative changes after the cessation of stressful events appeared to be an important factor in the onset of somatic disease.

Gellhorn (cited by Beck, 1972) has expressed the opinion that people differ in the degree of dominance of the sympathetic or the parasympathetic nervous system. His findings that the parasympathetic system dominated in PU patients, whereas the sympathetic system was dominant in persons with hypertension, correspond quite well with the results of the present study. The rise in SBP, DBP, and HR for MI patients in the stress situation is associated with sympathetic activity; the decline in these physiological measures found for the PU patients can be attributed to parasympathetic activity. It should be pointed out, however, that the pattern of emotional reactions observed in the present study was revealed only under stress. Therefore, research on the psychological determinants of the onset of somatic disease cannot be limited to situational or personality variables alone. The emotional reaction pattern arises from the interaction between these classes of variables (see, among others, Ress, 1983).

I am aware that the findings presented in this chapter and the concepts formulated on the basis of this research have a number of limitations. The subjects were tested in only one stress situation, overt behavior was not considered, and fragmented patterns of emotional reaction were studied, that is, only three physiological indicators and three measures of subjective emotional experience were used. Moreover, the study was retrospective and not prospective, only two groups of patients were evaluated, and these groups were small. Nevertheless, the results provide insight into how psychological factors may contribute to the onset and progression of somatic disease and may also have important implications for prevention, for example, the potential benefit of using biofeedback techniques with persons who experience highly persistent vegetative changes in response to stress.

In studies of the psychological determinants of the onset of somatic disease, investigation cannot be limited solely to personality or situational variables; an interactional model must necessarily be taken into account. In further research on emotional reactions to stressful situations, multiple physiological variables, measures of relevant emotional states, and overt behavioral variables should be recorded. The relation of emotional reaction patterns to the type of stressor situation should also be evaluated.

Because the resources for prospective research are lacking, other methods are being used to negate arguments that the findings reflect the effects, and not the causes, of somatic illness. For example, three groups of women are presently being studied: asthmatic patients, women whose limbs were amputated after an accident, and healthy persons. The postaccident patient group is considered a second control group on the assumption that the emotional reactions of these women had no influence on the onset of their infirmity. The relative independence of emotional reactions from the type of stress will be verified by exposing all subjects to two types of stressful situations, involving either physical or psychological threat. Finding differences in the emotional reactions of the asthmatic patients as compared with the controls, and no differences between the two control groups, would provide evidence of a relation between emotional reaction patterns and the onset of somatic disease.

In conclusion, the results of the present study support the hypothesis that people differ in their emotional reactions to stressful situations, and that the emotional reactions of persons afflicted with certain somatic illnesses differ from those of healthy persons. Differences in the emotional reaction patterns of persons afflicted with coronary heart disease and peptic ulcers were also found. Among these differences, the onset of somatic disease appears to be associated with the persistence of vegetative changes after the cessation of a stress situation.

SUMMARY

The relation between emotional reactions to stressful situations and the onset of somatic disease were investigated in three groups of 20 male, white-collar workers: Myocardial infarction and ulcer patients and persons in good health. All subjects responded to the Raven's Progressive Matrices Test in a threatening psychosocial situation. Emotional reaction patterns in a neutral situation, during a stressful experimental situation, and after the experiment were evaluated using Spielberger's three-factor STPI to measure anxiety, anger, and curiosity and systolic and diastolic blood pressure and heart rate to measure physiological changes. Significant differences were found between healthy and sick subjects and between myocardial infarction and ulcer patients on both psychological and physiological indicators.

REFERENCES

Aragon, A. (1970). *Dynamika reagowania na stres w etiologii choroby wrzodowej* [Dynamics of stress response and peptic ulcer etiology]. Unpublished master's thesis, University of Warsaw, Warszawa.

Beck, A. T. (1972). Cognition, anxiety and psychophysiological disorders. In C. D. Spielberger (Ed.), *Anxiety: Current trends in theory and research* (Vol. 2, pp. 343–354). New York: Academic Press.

Borkovec, T. M. (1976). Physiological and cognitive processes in the regulation of anxiety. In G. E. Schwartz & D. Shapiro (Eds.), *Consciousness and self-regulation: Advances in research* (Vol. 1, pp. 261–312). New York: Plenum Press.

Cameron, D. E. (1944). Observations on the patterns of anxiety. *American Journal of Psychiatry, 101*, 36.

Croog, H. C., & Levine, S. (1977). *The heart patient recovers: Sociological and psychological factors.* New York: Human Sciences Press.

Hackett, T. P., & Cassem, N. H. (1974). Development of a quantitative rating scale to assess denial. *Journal of Psychosomatic Research, 18*, 93.

Lacey, J. I., Bateman, D. E., & Van Lehn, R. (1953). Autonomic response specificity. *Psychosomatic Medicine, 15*, 8.

Lacey, J. I., & Lacey, B. C. (1958). Verification and extension of the principle of autonomic response stereotypy. *American Journal of Psychology, 71*, 50.

Lazowski, J. (Ed.). (1978). *Problemy psychosomatyczne w chorobie wrzodowej żołądka i dwunastnicy* [Psychosomatic problems of peptic ulcers]. Warsaw, Poland: PZWL.

Lepczyński, P. (1983). *Wzór reagowania fizjologicznego a choroba psychosomatyczna* [Physiological patterns and reactions and psychosomatic disease]. Unpublished master's thesis, University of Warsaw, Warszawa.

Mandler, G. Mandler, J. M., & Uviller, E. T. (1958). Autonomic feedback: The perception of autonomic activity. *Journal of Abnormal and Social Psychology, 56*, 367.

Pleszewski, Z. (1977). *Funkcjonowanie emocjonalne pacjentów przed i po zawale serca* [Emotional functioning of the patients before and after myocardial infarction]. Poznań, Poland: UAM.

Ress, L. (1983). The development of psychosomatic medicine during the past 25 years. *Journal of Psychosomatic Research, 27*, 157.

Reykowski, J., & Krawczyk, M. (1972). Emocje, osobowość a choroba psychosomatyczna [Emotion, personality, and psychosomatic disease]. *Psychologia Wychowawcza, 15*, 542.

Sosnowski, T., & Wrześniewski, K. (1983). Polska adaptacja Inwentarza STAI do badania stanu i cechy leku [Development of the Polish form of the STAI]. *Przeglad Psychologiczny, 26*, 2.

Spielberger, C. D. (1979). *Preliminary manual for the State-Trait Personality Inventory (STPI): Test forms and psychometric data.* Tampa, FL: University of South Florida.

Spielberger, C. D., Gorsuch, R. L., & Lushene, R. E. (1970). *Manual for the State-Trait Anxiety Inventory.* Palo Alto: Consulting Psychologists Press.

Steptoe, A. (1980). Stress and medical disorders. In S. Rachman (Ed.), *Contributions to medical psychology,* (Vol. 2, pp. 55–77). Oxford, England: Pergamon Press.

Valek, J., & Kuhn, E. (1970). Stress-induced changes of carbohydrate and lipid metabolism in coronary heart disease. In R. A. Pierloot (Ed.), *Recent research in psychosomatics.* Basel: Karger.

Wrześniewski, K. (1980). *Psychologiczne problemy chorych z zawałem serca* [Psychological problems of myocardial infarction patients]. Warsaw, Poland: PZWL.

Wrześniewski, K. (1984). Development of the Polish form of the State-Trait Personality Inventory. In H. M. van der Ploeg, R. Schwarzer, C. D. Spielberger (Eds.), *Advances in test anxiety research* (Vol. 3, pp. 265–275). Lisse, the Netherlands: Swets and Zeitlinger.

4

Coping with War Anxiety:
An Experimental Analysis

Philip A. Saigh
American University of Beirut, Lebanon

Although interest in posttraumatic stress disorder (PTSD) has waxed appreciably since America's involvement in Vietnam (Fairbank, Jarvie, & Keane, 1981; Silver, 1982), the essential features of this condition have been recorded for centuries. Herodotus provided an early account of the disorder following the Battle of Marathon in 490 B.C. (Rawlinson, 1893). A more personalized description of PTSD symptoms is evident in the 16th-century diary of Samuel Pepys. Writing 6 months after he witnessed the Great Fire of London, Pepys (1667/1974) observed that "it is strange to think how to this very day I cannot sleep a-night without great terrors of the fire."

In a similar vein, Southard chronicled the PTSD of a French corporal who witnessed the violent deaths of his comrades and who, in turn, was temporarily buried alive when his trench collapsed. Although the corporal escaped physical injury, "his pulse was variable; at rest it stood at 60; if a table nearby was struck suddenly, it would go up to 120" (Southard, 1919, p. 309). Similar descriptions of the mental status of the survivors of natural disasters (Adams & Adams, 1984; Burke, Borus, Burns, Millstein, & Beasley, 1982; Patrick & Patrick, 1981), accidents (Friedman & Linn, 1957; Glass, 1954; Green, Grace, Lindy, Titchner, & Lindy, 1983; Kasl, Chisholm, & Eskenazi, 1981), rape (Norris & Feldman, 1981; Vernon & Kilpatrick, 1980), and assault (Kinder, 1982; Siegal, 1983) have contributed to a conceptual synthesis with regard to the nature of PTSD.

According to the American Psychiatric Association's *Diagnostic and Statistical Manual of Mental Disorders* (*DSM-III*), PTSD is indicated by "the development of characteristic symptoms following a psychologically traumatic event that is generally outside the range of usual human experience (American Psychiatric Association [APA], 1980, p. 236). These symptoms typically involve high levels of anxiety, repeated thoughts about the trauma, blunted affect, and a number of specific behavioral manifestations such as exaggerated startle response, avoidance behaviors, and memory impairment. The *DSM-III* also states that "the disorder is apparently more severe and longer lasting when the stressor is of human design" (APA, 1980, p. 236). Finally, the *DSM-III* subdivides PTSD into two categories, namely, acute and chronic. Acute PTSD is indicated when "the symptoms begin within six months of the trauma and have not lasted six months" (APA, 1980, p. 237), whereas the

Philip A. Saigh is currently a professor at the Graduate School of the City University of New York.

chronic PTSD category is warranted "if the symptoms either develop more than six months after the trauma or last six months or more" (APA, 1980, p. 237).

From a different perspective, the ninth edition of the World Health Organization's (WHO) *International Classification of Diseases (ICD-9)* USDHHS, lists trauma-related symptomatology under the heading of stress reactions. As in the case of the APA's PTSD classification, the *ICD-9* subdivides stress reactions into two categories. The first category involves acute stress reactions that are described as "transient disorders of any severity and nature of emotions, consciousness, and psychomotor states . . . without pre-existing mental disorder in response to exceptional physical and mental stress such as combat or natural disasters or battle. . . ." (USDHHS, 1980, p. 1123). The *ICD-9* also indicates that acute stress reactions generally subside within hours or days of the trauma. The second *ICD-9* category involves adjustment reactions that are described as "lasting longer than acute stress reactions . . . relatively circumscribed . . . and . . . closely related in time and content" (USDHHS, 1980, p. 1078).

Considered from an epidemiological perspective, it is interesting to note that, despite the abundance of war-related stress studies (Babinski & Fromet, 1918; Bourne, 1970; Glass, 1954; Janis, 1951; Mitchell, Morehouse, & Keen, 1864; Richards, 1910), consensus with regard to the prevalence of PTSD is lacking. On the basis of a compelling analysis of the British psychiatric literature published during World War II, Rachman (1978) concluded,

> The great majority of the people endured the air raids extraordinarily well, contrary to the universal expectation of mass panic. Exposure to repeated bombings did not produce significant increases in psychiatric disorders. Although short lived fear reactions were common, surprisingly few persistent phobic reactions emerged. (p. 186)

In a similar vein, Kettner (1972) analyzed the service records of 1,086 Swedish United Nations (UN) troops who saw action during 1961 in the Congo (now Zaire) and observed that only 35 soldiers succumbed to combat exhaustion. Four years after the events that transpired in the Congo, Kettner obtained the postmilitary medical records of the Swedish combatants and compared them with the postmilitary records of 1,242 Swedes stationed in the Congo who had not been exposed to combat. His results revealed that "the combat veterans did not differ from the noncombat veterans in total morbidity or psychiatric morbidity after their UN service" (p. 98). Similarly, on the basis of an analysis of the medical records of American servicemen stationed in Vietnam, Bourne (1970) concluded that "the most significant finding of the conflict has been that the number of psychiatric casualties has been amazingly low" (pp. 124–125).

Despite the apparent consensus in the reports of Rachman, Kettner, and Bourne, a different conclusion was reached by Egendorf, Kadushin, Laufer, Rothbart, and Sloan (1981). These authors interviewed 1,089 Vietnam veterans and concluded that 16.6% of the overall sample of 29.6% of the interviewees with combat experience developed emotional problems after they were repatriated. In a similar study, Keane and Fairbank (1983) surveyed 1,380 mental health practitioners at 114 Veterans Administration medical centers across the United States and reported that "the most consistent finding of the survey was the rating of Vietnam veterans as more poorly adjusted than veterans of previous wars. . . ." (p. 350).

Given the epidemiological disparity, it is interesting to observe that divergent explanations have been formulated to account for PTSD. For example, Freud (1919) posited that

> War neuroses are to be regarded as traumatic neuroses whose occurrence has been made possible or has been prompted by a conflict in the ego. . . . The conflict is between the soldier's old peaceful ego and his new warlike one, and becomes acute as soon as the peace-ego realizes what chances it runs of loosing its life owing to the rashness of its newly formed parasitic double. (p. 85)

Horowitz and Solomon (1975) have proposed that PTSD is due to the operation of two natural processes, an

> intrusive-repetitive tendency and a denial numbing tendency . . . the former tendency is an automatic property of mental information processing which serves the functions of assimilation and accommodation. . . . The denial-numbing tendency is . . . a defense function that interrupts repetition-to-completion in order to ward off intolerable ideas and emotions. (pp. 68–69)

Kean, Fairbank, Caddell, Zimering, and Beviler (1985) developed a two-factor behavioral formulation which posits that

> Individuals who have experienced life-threatening trauma become conditioned to a wide assortment of stimuli present during the event. Other people present, the place, the time of day, and even cognitions become associated with anxiety from the event and are capable of evoking extremely high levels of arousal. (p. 263)

The majority of the war-related stress studies are either surveys (Keane & Fairbank, 1983; Kettner, 1972), case studies (Baider & Rosenfield, 1974; Levav, Greenfield, & Barush, 1979), or treatment-oriented reports (Black & Kean, 1982; Saigh, 1987). Most of these studies were conducted *after* people had been exposed to traumatic events. Consequently, information pertaining to how people may change over time as a function of puissant stress is very limited (Quarantelli, 1985). Because of justifiable ethical and legal constraints, psychologists cannot intentionally assess people's behavior before and after exposing them to an actual trauma. Occasionally, however, fate takes a hand in these matters and serendipitous natural experiments have enabled psychologists to observe people's behavior before and after they were exposed to an actual trauma. Such an opportunity presented itself to me through my work as a faculty member at the American University of Beirut (Saigh, 1984a, 1984b, 1985a, 1985b).

SUBJECTS AND BACKGROUND

During the spring of 1982, I was in the process of cross-validating a battery of self-report anxiety inventories. Within this context, 77 Lebanese students who were attending a West Beirut junior high school were assessed during the first week of April. Similarly, 128 Lebanese undergraduates enrolled at the American University of Beirut (also in West Beirut) were assessed during the last week of May.

On June 6, 1982 (57 days after the junior high school administration and 6 days after the undergraduate administration), Israel invaded Lebanon. By June 14, West Beirut was surrounded by Israeli units. Although a substantial number of West Beirut's civilians evacuated to safer locations, a number of civilians remained in

West Beirut throughout the 10-week siege. In the course of these events, the people who elected to remain in West Beirut were exposed to considerable shelling, strafing, and bombing. They also experienced profound physical hardship as their water and electricity were turned off and food, medicine, and petrol were in short supply.

Following the withdrawal of Israeli, Palestinian, and Syrian forces, the Lebanese government, with the aid of American, French, and Italian forces, was able to exert its authority over the capital for the first time in 7 years. Although the government's tenure of authority over West Beirut was limited to a 16-month period, the reassertion of Lebanese sovereignty was associated with a substantial reduction in the level of hostilities. The roads between the Christian and Moslem quarters of the city reopened and sniping, abductions, shelling, and the like stopped.

The author located 64 of the junior high school students who had been previously tested. Their mean age was 14.6 years with a standard deviation of 0.9 years. The mean IQ of these students, as measured by the Lebanese Intelligence Scale for Adults (Saigh, 1983), was 108 with a standard deviation of 12 units. Of the 64 students, 16 (11 boys and 5 girls) reported that they had not evacuated and 48 (27 boys and 21 girls) reported that they had evacuated to safer locations before the siege began. All of these students were reassessed 8 weeks after the opposing forces withdrew from Beirut. Six months after the disengagement, 46 junior high school evacuees (26 boys and 20 girls) and 16 nonevacuees (11 boys and 5 girls) were located and reassessed.

Similarly, 98 previously tested undergraduates were located 6 weeks after the disengagement. Their mean age was 20.6 years with a standard deviation of 2.5 years; the mean IQ of the undergraduates on the Lebanese Intelligence Scale for Adults was 125, with a standard deviation of 10 units. Of the total group, 38 (20 men and 18 women) reported that they had been in West Beirut throughout the summer and 50 (21 men and 29 women) said that they had left West Beirut less than 1 week after it was encircled by the Israelis, that is, before basic services were cut off and the start of the major hostilities. These students were reassessed during the first week of November 1982. Six months later, 35 undergraduate evacuees (15 men and 10 women) and 20 undergraduate nonevacuees (9 men and 11 women) were located and reassessed.

The tests administered were Saigh's (1982) Lebanese Fear Inventory (LFI), Wolpe and Lang's (1964) Fear Survey Schedule (FSS), and the Spielberger, Gorsuch, and Lushene (1970) State–Trait Anxiety Inventory (STAI). The LFI is a discrete index of situationally specific behaviors or events that could have led to death, injury, or prodigious emotional discomfort before Lebanese sovereignty was reestablished over the capital, for example, snipers, crossing from the "Christian" to the "Moslem" side of Beirut or vice versa (Saigh, 1982, p. 353). The FSS is a measure of specific fears that consists of a wide range of situationally specific, potentially anxiety-provoking items, for example, the prospect of a surgical operation, airplanes, medical odors, germs, and dogs (Wolpe & Lang, 1964, p. 28). The STAI is made up of a State Anxiety Scale that measures the amount of anxiety that the subject is experiencing at the time of testing and a Trait Anxiety Scale that measures individual differences in anxiety proneness. An analysis of the psychometric properties of these measures for Lebanese students has been presented elsewhere (Mathia, 1981; Mathia & Saigh, 1983; Saigh, 1983).

RESULTS

A series of analyses of variance revealed that the preinvasion scores on the LFI, FSS, and STAI of the junior high school evacuees were not significantly different from the preinvasion anxiety scores of their classmates who did not evacuate. Similar nonsignificant differences were noted between the preinvasion undergraduate evacuee and nonevacuee groups. No significant differences were evident between the postinvasion scores of the junior high school evacuees and nonevacuees. Also, no significant differences were found in the postinvasion scores of the undergraduate evacuees and nonevacuees.

The junior high school preinvasion, 8-week postinvasion, and 6-month postinvasion scores were compared by means of a Scheffé analysis. No significant differences were found on the FSS or STAI (State and Trait Anxiety Scales), but the LFI scores recorded 8 weeks and 6 months after the invasion were significantly lower than the preinvasion scores. There were no significant differences between the 8-week and 6-months postinvasion LFI scores. Similar results were found when the undergraduate preinvasion, 6-week postinvasion, and 6-month postinvasion scores were compared. A schematic presentation of the students' level of arousal is presented in Figures 1 and 2.

DISCUSSION

The results indicated that the self-reported anxiety levels of the junior high school and undergraduate respondents who remained in West Beirut closely corresponded to the level of anxiety of their counterparts who evacuated. The results

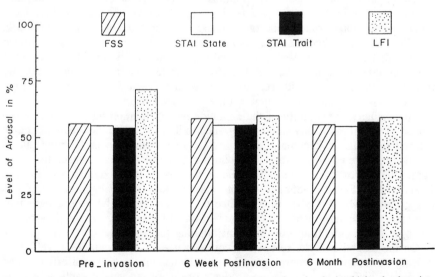

Figure 1 Preinvasion, 8 weeks postinvasion, and 6 months postinvasion junior high school anxiety estimates (FSS = Fear Survey Schedule, STAI = State–Trait Anxiety Inventory, LFI = Lebanese Fear Inventory).

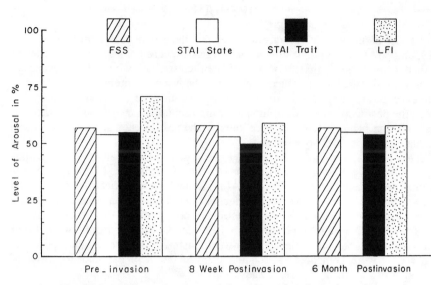

Figure 2 Preinvasion, 6 weeks postinvasion, and 6 months postinvasion undergraduate anxiety estimates (FSS = Fear Survey Schedule, STAI = State–Trait Anxiety Inventory, LFI = Lebanese Fear Inventory).

also suggested that the respondents' level of arousal vis-à-vis war-related stimuli was markedly lower at postassessment.

These observations are largely incompatible with the conditioning theory of fear acquisition (Mowrer, 1939; Rachman, 1978; Seligman & Hagen, 1972), which implicitly holds that any stimulus can become a conditioned stimulus through association (i.e., the equipotentiality premise). On the basis of these theoretical assumptions, some of the situationally specific items that make up the FSS or LFI should have been associated with the aversive events (i.e., unconditioned stimuli) that occurred in West Beirut, and these associations should have resulted in higher anxiety ratings. The fact that this did not happen, along with the nonsignificant STAI results, would seem to raise questions regarding the validity of the conditioning formulation as it applies to war-induced fears.

Conceptually, the validity of the conditioning formulation has also been challenged by aversion therapy studies that failed to induce conditioned fears in human subjects (Hallman & Rachman, 1976), and by the results of social learning studies that demonstrated that human fear reactions may be vicariously transmitted (Bandura, 1980). Moreover, the efficacy of exposure-based PTSD treatments (Black & Keane, 1982; Saigh, 1985c) does not support the conditioning model, as was suggested by Marks (1981, p. 8): "One cannot argue that because a particular treatment is effective for a particular condition, it necessarily throws light on the etiology of that condition or even its maintaining factors."

On the other hand, the results are commensurate with Bandura's (1980) self-efficacy formulation. According to this conceptualization, personal efficacy and the degree of fear arousal are the products of the reciprocal interaction between previous learning, the perceived ability to perform specific acts (e.g., driving from the Christian to the Moslem quarter of Beirut), and the anticipated outcomes (consequences) of engaging in or experiencing the behaviors or events that make up the LFI. Given that the LFI reflects situational motifs that could have led to death, injury, or considerable emotional discomfort before and during the invasion, and because the situational factors that maintained these fears were reduced or eliminated after law and order was reestablished in the capital, it may be argued that the respondents were less anxious because they *knew* that the negative contingencies that had regulated their behavior were no longer present.

These comments should be tempered with the realization that a number of factors may have influenced the validity of the preinvasion and postinvasion conclusions. Specifically, the Lebanese data were based exclusively on self-reports, and these indices may have served "instrumentally to achieve other anticipated consequences for individuals, leading to responses that are simply untrue and that depend on the individual's assessment of the situation" (Borkovec, Weerts, & Bernstein, 1977, p. 405). Moreover, information pertaining to the respondents' level of physiological arousal and overt behavioral data were not collected. The validity of the findings may also have been affected by attrition as a number of the initial respondents could not be located for reassessment. Finally, because the naturalistic design of the study precluded random assignment of subjects to groups, the subjective experiences of the respondents could not be controlled.

Nevertheless, the findings of this study are consistent with the epidemiological conclusions that were independently reached by Rachman (1978), Kettner (1972), and Bourne (1970), and with recent reports of the favorable psychological adjustment of British bomb disposal units in Northern Ireland (Hallman, 1983). Accordingly, it appears that prolonged exposure to life-threatening events that are subsequently mollified may not induce higher levels of anxiety at a later date. Moreover, situation-specific, self-reported anxiety may decrease following the withdrawal of the stimuli that initially mediated these fears.

FUTURE DIRECTIONS

There is a considerable need to arrive at a clearer understanding of the prevalence and correlates of PTSD. The discordant theoretical formulations that have been proposed introduce confusion and ambiguity that may influence the scope and course of the treatment modalities that are being developed (Saigh, 1985c). Although extant theories offer provocative speculations about the etiology of the disorder, for the time being it may be more appropriate to forego etiological theorization and concentrate on more substantive research. Within this context there is a need to develop a standardized battery of tests to reflect the multiple parameters of PTSD. The singular use of projective tests, polygraphs, behavioral avoidance tests, and anxiety inventories can only serve to provide a partial description of the disorder.

It is encouraging to note that Fairbank, Keane, and Malloy (1983) established the discriminate validity of a PTSD test battery with a small sample of adult patients, and it is hoped that additional research with larger samples will corroborate their results. Similar research should also be directed toward the validation of PTSD assessment packages for children, as there is a notable dearth of information pertaining to the assessment of childhood PTSD.

Research can also be facilitated by more detailed sample descriptions of PTSD patients (cf. Escobar et al., 1983); vague sample descriptions have contributed to difficulties in formulating viable generalizations about the disorder. Similarly, the development of an operational definition for the term *significant stress* would be useful in reducing the degree of contention that has arisen over the use of this construct (Saigh, 1985c). A more precise and quantified definition would reduce trauma-related diagnostic errors.

It would also be appropriate to use multiple research approaches in order to obtain a clearer understanding of war-related stress. The utility of this approach was recently demonstrated in a study that examined the course of anxiety, depression, and assertion before, during, and after a circumscribed war trauma (Saigh, 1988). The group data from this study revealed that the scores recorded during the traumatic interval significantly differed from the scores recorded before and after the trauma, but no significant differences were observed between the pretrauma and posttrauma scores. When a single-case analysis (Barlow & Hersen, 1984) was subsequently conducted, it became evident that some of the respondents developed and maintained symptomatology that was suggestive of PTSD following the trauma. Although the between-groups and single-case analyses yielded singular information, a more meaningful and comprehensive account emerged when the results were viewed in concert.

Finally, it is essential to determine why some people develop PTSD and why others do not, given similar traumatic exposures. Information of this sort would facilitate a conceptual synthesis with regard to the nature of the disorder and contribute to developing more comprehensive and effective treatment programs.

REFERENCES

Adams, P. P., & Adams, G. R. (1984). Mount Saint Helens's ashfall: Evidence for a disaster stress reaction. *American Psychologist, 39,* 252–260.

American Psychiatric Association. (1980). *Diagnostic and statistical manual of mental disorders* (3rd ed.). Washington, DC: Author.

Babinski, J., & Fromet, J. (1918). *Hysteria and pithiatism.* London: University of London Press.

Baider, L., & Rosenfield, E. (1974, October). Effect of parental fears on children in wartime. *Social Work,* 497–502.

Bandura, A. (1980). Reflections on self-efficacy. In C. M. Franks & G. T. Wilson (Eds.), *Annual review of behavior therapy and practice 1979.* New York: Brunner/Mazel.

Barlow, D. H., & Hersen, M. (1984). *Single-case experimental design: Strategies for studying behavior change* (2nd ed.). New York: Pergamon Press.

Black, J. L., & Keane, T. M. (1982). Implosive therapy in the treatment of combat related fears in a World War II veteran. *Journal of Behaviour Therapy and Experimental Psychiatry, 13,* 163–165.

Borkovec, T., Weerts, T., & Bernstein, M. (1977). The assessment of anxiety. In A. Ciminero, K. Calhoun, & H. Adams (Eds.), *Handbook of behavioral assessment* (pp. 367–428). New York: Brunner/Mazel.

Bourne, P. J. (1970). Military psychiatry and the Vietnam experience. *American Journal of Psychiatry, 127,* 481–488.

Burke, J. D., Borus, J. F., Burns, B. J., Millstein, K. H., & Beasley, M. C. (1982). Changes in children's behavior after a natural disaster. *American Journal of Psychiatry, 139,* 1010–1014.

Egendorf, A., Kadushin, R. S., Laufer, R. S., Rothbart, G., & Sloan, L. (1981). *Legacies of Vietnam: Comparative adjustment of veterans and their peers.* New York: Center for Policy Research.

Escobar, J. I., Randolph, E. T., Puente, G., Spiwak, F., Asamen, J. K., Hill, M. H., & Hough, R. L. (1983). Post-traumatic stress disorder in Hispanic Vietnam veterans: Clinical phenomenology and social characteristics. *Journal of Nervous and Mental Diseases, 171,* 585–596.

Fairbank, J. A., Jarvie, G. J., & Keane, T. M. (1981). A selected bibliography of posttraumatic stress disorders in Vietnam veterans. *Professional Psychology, 12,* 578–610.

Fairbank, J. A., Keane, T. M., & Malloy, P. F. (1983). Some preliminary data on the psychological characteristics of Vietnam veterans with post-traumatic stress disorder. *Journal of Consulting and Clinical Psychology, 51,* 912–919.

Freidman, P., & Linn, L. (1957). Some psychiatric notes on the Andrea Doria disaster. *American Journal of Psychiatry, 114,* 426–432.

Freud, S. (1919). Psycho-analysis and war neuroses. In J. Strachey (Ed.), *Sigmund Freud, M.D., LL.D.: Collected papers* (Vol. 5, p. 5). London: Hogarth Press.

Glass, A. J. (1954). Psychotherapy in the combat zone. *American Journal of Psychiatry, 10,* 578–586.

Green, B. L., Grace, M. C., Lindy, J. D., Titchner, J. L., & Lindy, J. G. (1983). Levels of functional impairment following a civilian disaster: The Beverly Hills supper club fire. *Journal of Consulting and Clinical Psychology, 50,* 573–580.

Hallman, R. S. (1983). Psychometric analysis. *Advances in Behaviour Research and Therapy, 4,* 105–120.

Hallman, R. S., & Rachman, S. (1976). Current status of aversion therapy. In M. Hersen, R. Eisler, & P. Miller (Eds.), *Progress in behavior modification* (Vol. 2, pp. 179–219). New York: Academic Press.

Horowitz, M. J., & Solomon, G. F. (1975). A prediction of delayed stress response syndromes in Vietnam veterans. *Journal of Social Issues, 31,* 67–80.

Janis, I. (1951). *Air war and emotional stress.* New York: McGraw-Hill.

Kasl, S. V., Chisholm, R. F., & Eskenazi, B. (1981). The impact of the accident at Three Mile Island on the behavior and well being of nuclear workers. *American Journal of Public Health, 71,* 472–495.

Keane, T. M., & Fairbank, J. A. (1983). Survey analysis of combat-related stress disorders in Vietnam veterans. *American Journal of Psychiatry, 140,* 348–350.

Keane, T. M., Fairbank, J. A., Caddell, J. M., Zimering, R. T., & Beviler, M. E. (1985). A behavioral approach to assessing and treating posttraumatic stress disorder in Vietnam veterans. In C. R. Figley (Ed.), *Trauma and its wake* (pp. 257–294). New York: Brunner/Mazel.

Kettner, B. (1972). Combat strain and subsequent mental health. *Acta Psychiatrica Scandinavica, 22,* 5–107.

Kinder, G. (1982). *Victim: The other side of murder.* New York: Delacorte Press.

Levav, I., Greenfield, H., & Barush, E. (1979). Psychiatric combat reactions during the Yom Kippur War. *American Journal of Psychiatry, 136,* 637–641.

Marks, I. (1981). *Cure and care of neuroses.* New York: Wiley.

Mathia, M. (1981). *Lebanese norms for the Fear Survey Schedule.* Unpublished master's thesis, American University of Beirut.

Mathia, M., & Saigh, P. A. (1983, December). *Lebanese psychometric data for the Fear Survey Schedule.* Paper presented at the meeting of the World Congress of Behavior Therapy, Washington, DC.

Mitchell, S. W., Morehouse, C. R., & Keen, W. S. (1864). *Gunshot wounds and other injuries of the nerves.* Philadelphia, PA: Lippincott.

Mowrer, O. H. (1939). Stimulus response theory of anxiety. *Psychological Review, 46,* 553–565.

Norris, J., & Feldman, S. S. (1981). Factors related to the psychological impact of rape on the victim. *American Journal of Abnormal Psychology, 90,* 562–567.

Patrick, R. W., & Patrick, W. K. (1981). Cyclone '78 in Srilanka: The mental health trail. *British Journal of Psychiatry, 138,* 210–216.

Pepys, S. (1974). The diary of Samuel Pepys. In R. Latham & W. Mathews (Eds.), *The diary of Samuel Pepys* (pp. 1–450). Los Angeles: University of California Press. (Original work published 1667)

Quarantelli, E. L. (1985). An assessment of conflicting views on mental health: The consequences of traumatic events. In C. R. Figley (Ed.), *Trauma and its wake* (pp. 173–218). New York: Brunner/Mazel.

Rachman, S. (1978). *Fear and courage.* San Francisco: Freeman.

Rawlinson, G. C. (1893). *The history of Herodotus.* New York: Appleton.

Richards, P. L. (1910). Mental and nervous disease in the Russo-Japanese War. *Military Surgery, 26,* 177–193.

Saigh, P. A. (1982). The Lebanese Fear Inventory: A normative report. *Journal of Clinical Psychology, 38,* 352–355.

Saigh, P. A. (1983). *The Lebanese Intelligence Scale for Adults.* Beirut, Lebanon: Privately printed.

Saigh, P. A. (1984a). An experimental analysis of delayed posttraumatic stress. *Behaviour Research and Therapy, 22,* 679–682.

Saigh, P. A. (1984b). Pre- and postinvasion anxiety in Lebanon. *Behavior Therapy, 15,* 185–190.

Saigh, P. A. (1985a). Adolescent anxiety following varying degrees of war stress in Lebanon. *Journal of Clinical Child Psychology, 14,* 210–215.

Saigh, P. A. (1985b). An experimental analysis of delayed posttraumatic stress among adolescents. *Journal of Genetic Psychology, 146,* 125–131.

Saigh, P. A. (1985c). On the nature and etiology of traumatic stress. *Behavior Therapy, 16,* 423–426.

Saigh, P. A. (1987). In vitro flooding of an adolescent posttraumatic stress disorder. *Journal of Clinical Child Psychology, 16,* 147–150.

Saigh, P. A. (1988). Anxiety, depression, and assertion across alternating intervals of war. *Journal of Abnormal Psychology, 97,* 338–341.

Seligman, M., & Hagen, J. (1972). *Biological boundries of learning.* New York: Appleton-Century-Crofts.

Siegal, M. (1983). Crime and violence in America. *American Psychologist, 38,* 1267–1273.

Silver, S. M. (1982). Posttraumatic stress disorders in Vietnam veterans: An addendum to Fairbank et al. *Professional Psychology, 13,* 522–525.

Southard, E. E. (1919). *Shell shock and neuropsychiatric problems.* Boston: Leonard.

Spielberger, C. D., Gorsuch, R. L., & Lushene, R. E. (1970). *Manual for the State–Trait Anxiety Inventory.* Palo Alto, CA: Consulting Psychologists Press.

United States Department of Health and Human Services. (1980). *The international classification of diseases 9th revision: Clinical modification.* (DHHS Publication No. (PHS) 80-1260). Washington, DC: U.S. Government Printing Office.

Vernon, L. J., & Kilpatrick, D. G. (1980). Self-reported fears of rape victims: A preliminary report. *Behavior Modification, 4,* 383–396.

Wolpe, J., & Lang, P. (1964). A Fear Survey Schedule for use in behavior therapy. *Behaviour Research and Therapy, 2,* 27–30.

5

Self-Esteem, Realization of Life Purposes, and Level of Anxiety in Aged Persons

Ivan G. Paspalanov
University of Sofia, Bulgaria

Research on anxiety in elderly persons and the development of measures of anxiety in this age group have received relatively little attention. Although specialized anxiety scales have been constructed for children and adults, many of the items in such scales may not be appropriate for older-aged groups. Moreover, during the process of aging, some anxiety symptoms may be reduced and others may occur more often or have heightened influence. Therefore, it seems essential to determine if anxiety symptoms in older people differ from those of younger persons.

The theoretical rationale for the development of trait anxiety as contrasted with state anxiety (see Spielberger, 1966, 1972a, 1972b, 1976) is based on the assumption that negative emotional experiences are evoked by life stress (Goldstein, 1939; Imedadze, 1966; Lader, 1972; Levitov, 1969; Mandler & Watson, 1966; May, 1950; Rogers, 1951). Consequently, in studying changes in anxiety as a function of age, it seems useful to examine the history of "dangerous stimuli" in broad general categories, such as frustration of basic life goals, unfulfilled aspirations, life crises, and so forth. Clarification of the relation between level of trait anxiety and specific life experiences will also enrich the understanding of trait anxiety as a basic psychological concept.

In modern gerontopsychological research, several relatively independent aspects of anxiety have been examined. First, anxiety is considered to be an important indicator of change in the emotional sphere for an aging individual. Several studies have reported a higher level of anxiety in aged persons (e.g., Whitbourne, 1976), but others have found no relation between age and anxiety. For example, in a study of 1,250 elderly people ranging in age from 55–75 years old, McDonald (1980) found significant age-related differences in life satisfaction, depressive mood, and rigidity, but no differences in anxiety level between age groups. The contradictory results in studies of anxiety in elderly persons may be partly due to the use of different methods to measure anxiety. Therefore, one of the primary goals of the present study was to develop scales suited for different age groups based on the same anxiety construct and with similar item content.

Botwinick (1973) interpreted anxiety in elderly populations as an Adjustment factor, which he used to explain behavioral manifestations that are typical of elderly persons, for example, risk avoidance, heightened cautiousness, lack of confidence, anticipation and fear of failure, and a general sense of uncertainty. In

Botwinick's opinion, the cautiousness of older persons and their eagerness for more information is due both to a decline in cognitive functioning, which is typical of the aging process, and to individual differences in anxiety as a personality trait. Anxiety in aged persons is assumed by many to be a basic parameter of personal adjustment, along with experiences of satisfaction and happiness, flexibility, self-concept, and the ability to endure psychological stress (Kuhlen, 1959).

In the emotional sphere of older persons, symptoms of depression have been examined mainly within a psychopathological framework, with the emphasis on brain neuropathology and physiological aging. On the other hand, emotional stability and a sense of happiness are generally associated with the entire course of the individual's life, that is, his or her social status and interpersonal interactions. Ignat Petrov (1978, p. 43), a Bulgarian gerontopsychologist, has stated

> Emotional stability is closely related to . . . "mental health". By "mental health" we mean not only the absence of a mental disturbance but also a most favourable and harmonious development of the individual throughout his life, giving him optimal opportunities of socially useful and creative activity.

Applying this approach in the study of anxiety in elderly people, it follows that level of anxiety can be influenced by overall success in life adjustment and the degree to which an individual has attained his or her basic life goals.

The goals of the present study[1] were as follows: (a) to study age and gender differences in the anxiety level of adults and older people living in their own homes or in special homes for the elderly; (b) to investigate the relation between anxiety and selected parameters of overall emotional status in this age group; (c) to examine the extent to which attaining one's life goals influences level of anxiety; and (d) to determine the relation between anxiety and the social characteristics of elderly persons, such as marital status, education, work and economic status, and social and sports activities.

METHOD

From the population of individuals of pensionable age,[2] 412 subjects were selected. Of these, 214 (96 men and 118 women) lived in their own homes and 198 (79 men and 119 women) were residents in homes for the elderly. The distribution of subjects from various social groups was approximately the same for both sexes. The following instruments were administered to all subjects:

1. *Trait Anxiety Scale*—This scale was developed for individuals more than 50 years of age on the basis of the Taylor (1953) Manifest Anxiety Scale. It contained 30 anxiety items and 10 distracting questions. The development of anxiety scales for different age groups is discussed later.

2. *Sociopsychological Questionnaire*—The Sociopsychological Questionnaire

---

[1]The investigation reported here is part of a representative social-psychological study on persons of pensionable age from Sofia that was carried out in 1980 by a research team headed by Professor G. Yolov. The study included 1,261 subjects; 884 of them (385 men and 499 women) lived in their own homes, whereas 377 individuals (129 men and 248 women) resided in special homes for the aged, supported by the state.

[2]The pensionable age for women in Bulgaria is 55; for men it is 60.

contains items related to job satisfaction, work aspirations, leisure activities, interpersonal interactions, immediate and long-term goals, value orientation, attitude toward family and relatives, the morality and industry of the younger generation, and other sociological indicators. The following subscales and items from the Sociopsychological Questionnaire were analyzed in the present study:

1. Five-point self-evaluation rating scale for general physical status as compared with other people of the same age ("much better than that of others," "on the whole, better than that of others," "same as that of others," "on the whole, worse than that of others," "much worse than that of others").

2. Three-point self-evaluation rating scale for adjustment to age-related psychological changes (in perception, memory, etc.; "I have noticed no special changes," "I have noticed some changes but they do not affect my self-confidence," "I have noticed some changes that definitely affect my self-confidence").

3. Three-point rating scale for recording feelings of adults and elderly people about the future ("with absolute confidence and certainty," "with some uneasiness," "with great uneasiness"). Lader's (1972) term, *prospective feeling*, is used to refer to these views about the future.

4. Three-point rating scales for assessing the degree to which individuals have attained their life purposes ("fully attained," "attained to a certain extent," "not attained at all") in the following five spheres: economic security, academic studies, profession, family and children, social activity.

The first three scales, namely, Physical Self-Confidence (PhSC), Adjustment to Psychological Change (APCh), and Anxiety Prospective Feelings (APF), were assumed to constitute the basic parameters of general self-confidence for adult and elderly persons. Finally, two open-ended questions were included to identify factors that determine prospective anxiety feelings and a sense of confidence and certainty ("What causes your uneasiness about the future?").

Development of Trait Anxiety Scale for Different Age Groups

Research began in 1978 on the adaptation and standardization of the Taylor (1953) Manifest Anxiety Scale (MAS) for the Bulgarian population.[3] Five bilingual specialists in psychology translated the scale items, reaching a consensus on the Bulgarian translation of each item. The translated items were evaluated in terms of content, meaning, and clarity of expression by 40 psychologists and psychology undergraduates who were fluent in English.

The preliminary Bulgarian MAS was administered to 100 male and 100 female students. An item analysis indicated that about half of the items did not meet the reliability criterion. Eight items with low reliability were eliminated at this early stage because about 25% of the subjects did not respond to them. Five of these items asked about physiological and vegetative disorders (diarrhea, constipation,

---

[3]This section was written in collaboration with Dimitar Stetinsky, head of a research group on improving psychological experiments at the Central Psychology Laboratory of the Bulgarian Academy of Sciences.

blushing, sweating). The items found not to be sufficiently reliable were rewritten so that they would be more acceptable.

Because a number of items assessed the same phenomena (e.g., there were three items for blushing), the unreliable items were eliminated, leaving two items for stomach troubles and one each for blushing, sweating, tearfulness, palpitation, and shortness of breath. The experts recommended that the eliminated items *not* be replaced by items in the physiological-vegetative sphere because normal subjects seemed reluctant to respond to such questions. With the experts' assistance, the following eight new items were formulated to assess various aspects of trait anxiety:

1. I often have doubts about my professional and academic success.
2. After emotional strain I often feel totally shaken.
3. I often do not feel steady enough.
4. I am very anxious to know what other people think of me.
5. I frequently feel uncertain.
6. I often have doubts about my capacity to work.
7. I can control myself most of the time.
8. When I learn that I have been talked about, my first thought is that I have been spoken ill of.

Before beginning the second stage of the standardization, another major problem had to be addressed: the addition of items in a manner that preserved the essential content of the trait anxiety construct. For this purpose, an assessment by experts and a qualitative analysis were carried out. Seven major groups of items having common qualities were identified and empirically verified by hierarchical cluster analysis (Johnson, 1967). The resulting dendograms proved almost identical for both groups of 100 subjects. The empirically established clusters validated the qualitative analysis and led to further elaboration of certain categories. The cluster analysis revealed a relatively stable structure for the anxiety items (Paspalanov & Stetinsky, 1980a, 1980b; Stetinsky & Paspalanov, 1980), allowing a qualitative definition of the clusters as follows.

1. *Neuroticism.* These items described emotional strain and nervousness ("I am a very nervous person," "I work under a great deal of strain"). It should be noted, however, that this group of items did not exhaust Eysenck's (1970) wider concept of neuroticism.

2. *Sensitivity and embarrassment.* Although similar to the first group of items, the common quality of these items was emotional sensitivity and embarrassment, for example, "I am easily embarrassed," "My feelings are hurt easier than most people's."

3. *Worries.* These items constituted two distinct subgroups: (a) *object-related worries*—worries about eventual failure, work, negative evaluations, and the like; (b) *diffuse worries*—for example, "I often catch myself worrying about something," "At times I have been worried beyond reason about something that really did not matter," "I worry about something or someone almost all the time."

4. *Lack of self-confidence and uncertainty.* These items imply lack of confidence in one's own abilities and feelings of uncertainty when undertaking any kind of activity ("I am not confident of myself at all," "I often have doubts about my

professional and academic success," "I have often felt that I faced so many difficulties I could not overcome them").

5. *Negative self-concept, complexes.* The self-concept items pertain to feelings of inferiority, being unable to cope with difficulties, and a sense of ineptitude and uselessness ("At times I think I am no good at all," "I certainly feel useless at times"). The items relating to negative complexes reflect the individual's self-concept and general outlook on life ("I wish I could be as happy as others").

6. *Activity regulation and work efficiency.* These items involve psychic regulation of activity and especially work efficiency, for example, exhaustion, concentration, general efficiency ("I frequently notice my hand shakes when I try to do something," "I find it hard to keep my mind on a task or job").

7. *Regulative and physiological symptoms.* Included here are items that assess the influence of chronic anxiety on an individual's behavior and general physiological status. Three subgroups can be differentiated: (a) *sleep characteristics*—restless and disturbed sleep, nightmares; (b) *physiological and vegetative symptoms*—breathlessness, palpitation, stomach troubles, headache, sweating, sickness—many of which are due to inborn physiological and nervous regulatory predispositions that, when reinforced by anxiety, develop into chronic symptoms (Lader, 1972); (c) *behavioral characteristics*—restlessness, lack of self-control, instability. Combined with chronic anxiety, these symptoms develop into unstable neurotic and behavioral traits ("It makes me nervous to have to wait," "At times I am so restless that I cannot sit in a chair for very long").

A concern in the second stage of scale development was that certain trait anxiety items established by cluster analysis would disappear if the low-reliability items were eliminated. The modified scale, including 30 distracting items, was administered to 800 subjects (400 men and 400 women) who were assigned to four age groups: 16–20, 21–30, 31–40, and 41–50 years old. The reliability of the items, and of the scale as a whole, was evaluated for both sexes in separate analyses for each age group. Because low reliability of an item might be due to either high or low marginals or low point-biserial coefficients, Gulliksen's formula (1950) was applied to the distributions and the marginal for each item. The results for this second stage of the psychometric analysis resulted in the identification of four groups of items:

1. *Items of low reliability in all age groups for both sexes.* Ten items are included in this group. Five of them owe their low reliability to their very low marginals, that is, very few subjects answer according to the key. Two additional items had very high marginals. The remaining 3 items had average marginals, but very low point-biserial correlations.

Eliminating these 10 items would not distort any of the differentiated clusters; each cluster would continue to comprise 4 items. The resulting briefer scale was more reliable and preserved the content of the trait anxiety construct.

2. *Items of high reliability in all age groups for both sexes.* These items were the most stable manifestations of trait anxiety, being valid for all age groups and not affected by gender. There were 15 items in this group, comprising primarily the categories of neuroticism and emotional strain, sleep characteristics, diffuse worries, lack of self-confidence and uncertainty, and activity control and work efficiency.

3. *Items whose reliability was determined by gender.* Of the 10 items in this category, 5 had high reliability for men of all age groups but were unreliable for women: "I worry very much about what other people think of me," "I worry over money and business," "I often find myself worrying about something," "I am more self-conscious than most people," "When I learn that I have been talked about, my first thought is I have been spoken ill of." The other 5 items had high reliability for women of all age groups, but were unreliable for men: "I am very confident of myself," "I cry easily," "I often notice my heart pounding and I am often short of breath," "I have very few headaches," and "I can control myself most of the time."

Psychometric analysis of these 10 items produced the following picture. Items with low reliability for men have average or slightly lower mean values and very low marginals. Thus, men were not likely to endorse the characteristics implied by these items, namely tearfulness, headaches, palpitation and shortness of breath, lack of self-confidence, and so forth. On the other hand, items with low reliability for women had low mean values, but average to high marginals. Thus, women having low levels of trait anxiety readily attributed the characteristics implied by these items to themselves.

4. *Items whose reliability was determined by age.* The item reliability analysis as a function of age revealed differences between two age ranges: 16–30 years old versus 31–50 years old. Four items were reliable for men and women in only one of these age groups, but unreliable for the other. For example, "I am happy most of the time" was reliable only for persons more than 30 years old, whereas "I find it hard to keep my mind on a task or job" was reliable only for the under-30 age groups.

5. *Items whose reliability was both gender- and age-determined.* The remaining items were unreliable for only one of the age ranges for men, but were reliable for women of both age ranges, or vice versa. Thus, the reliability of these items was affected by both gender- and age-related characteristics.

On the basis of the preceding analysis, the MAS, as standardized for the Bulgarian population from age 16 to 50 years, had a 15-item core. The reliability of these core items did not differ across age groups and was not affected by gender. However, a scale consisting of only 15 items was not considered adequate because the underlying construct validity of the original scale might be altered. Therefore, four differentiated scales were developed, respectively, for men and women belonging to the two age groups (16–30 and 31–50). In addition to the 15 core items, each scale included the 10 items found to be highly reliable for either men or women of one age group, plus the 5 items that were reliable for either men or women. The 30 items in the differentiated scales quite adequately represented all basic categories of the trait anxiety construct, as defined by cluster analysis.

In the first stage of this research, it was determined that 30 distracting questions were too many for the elderly subjects; they became tired and bored with responding to a 60-item scale. Therefore, in the second stage, the distracting questions were reduced to 14; the final scale consisted of 44 items. In the third stage of the present study, the four versions of the Anxiety scale were found to have excellent psychometric properties, as can be seen in Table 1. Special norms (*T* values) were developed for each age group for both sexes. The items constituting the four versions of the Anxiety scale are listed in Appendix A.

Table 1 Means, Standard Deviations, and Consistency Reliability Coefficients for the Scales in Different Sex and Age Groups

	Men				Women			
Age	N	M	SD	R	N	M	SD	R
16–20	100	12.20	5.80	.84	100	14.62	5.74	.84
21–30	100	13.00	6.11	.84	100	15.20	6.66	.84
31–40	100	13.22	6.21	.88	100	16.00	6.67	.86
41–50	100	14.20	6.41	.90	100	16.63	6.30	.85

DEVELOPMENT OF ANXIETY SCALE FOR ADULT AND AGED PERSONS

Following the strategy detailed in the preceding section, an Anxiety scale suitable for testing adults and older people was developed. The scales for 31- to 50-year-old men and women were administered to samples of 50 men and 50 women between 55–70 years of age. Item analyses showed that the following two items had low reliability for both women and men: "I often have doubts about my professional success" and "I often worry about failures that may come to me." In addition to poor reliability, the content of these items suggested that they were not suitable for people of pensionable age. With the help of five expert psychologists, two new items were formulated that appeared to be suitable for older men and women: "I often worry if I shall be able to cope with the problems the future might bring" and "I think (or worry) over the health of my relatives all the time."

Three additional items proved unreliable for men: "I often worry over money and business," "My feelings are hurt easier than most people's," and "I blush easily." On the basis of expert assessment, these items were replaced with the following three items that had high reliability for women over 55: "I have often felt that I faced so many difficulties I could not overcome them," "I am not at all confident of myself," and "I can control myself most of the time." Although these items had low reliability for younger men, we hypothesized that they would be appropriate for older men.

The findings in the second stage, in which samples of 100 men and 100 women over 50 years old were tested, were entirely positive: The two new items had high reliability coefficients for both men and women, and the three items that were initially reliable for women were found to be highly reliable for the older men. Table 2 reports the means, standard deviations, and reliability coefficients for men and women. The high reliability coefficients of both scales provided sufficient justification for using them to measure anxiety in younger and older adults. The scales for older men and women are presented in Appendix C and Appendix D.[4]

GENDER- AND AGE-RELATED DIFFERENCES IN ANXIETY

The means, standard deviations, and t tests of differences on the Anxiety scale for men and women residing in their own homes and in homes for the aged are

[4]These two scales, as well as the scales for younger age groups, may be used by researchers without obtaining the permission of the author or publisher.

Table 2 Means, Standard Deviations, and Consistency Reliability Coefficients for the Scales in the
Age Groups over 50

Sex	N	M	SD	R
Male	96	13.86	7.86	.80
Female	100	14.72	7.94	.85

presented in Table 3. The means for both groups were similar to the standardization sample (see Table 2). The older subjects were not higher in anxiety than
subjects under 50 years of age; indeed, the scores for subjects residing in their
own homes were lower for both men and women (compare with Table 1). Therefore, the results of the present study do not support McDonald's (1980) findings of
higher anxiety in aged persons.

The anxiety means for persons living in their own homes and those residing in
homes for the aged were not significantly different. Although some differences
were noted between the means for men and women (e.g., they were larger for the
sample residing in the homes for the aged), the *t* values were not statistically
significant. There was also a difference between the dispersions of item scores in
the over-50 age group and those 40–50 years old. Assessed by the *F* criterion for
dispersion comparison, this difference was statistically significant for both men
($p < .005$) and women ($p < .001$). This result was consistent with previous
findings that individual differences are greater in older age groups (Petrov, 1978).

CORRELATIONS BETWEEN ANXIETY AND SELF-ESTEEM

Anxiety scores were correlated with various parameters of overall self-esteem,
separately for male and female subjects who were divided into high-, medium-,
and low-anxiety groups. The anxiety scores for the subjects in these groups were
correlated with the self-esteem measures after calculating the "hi-square" criterion. Table 4 presents the correlations among the separate parameters of self-
esteem, as well as between these measures and level of anxiety.

The moderate negative correlations between LA on the one hand and PhSC and
APCh on the other (which were found for both adults and older people) can be

Table 3 Means, Standard Deviations, and Coefficients of Comparison on Anxiety for Men and
Women of both Samples

Groups	Men			Women			
	N	M	SD	N	M	SD	t
Group 1	96	13.24	7.21	118	14.12	7.52	0.86
Group 2	79	13.97	7.04	119	15.35	6.62	1.79
t		0.67			1.34		

Note. Group 1 = group of subjects living in their own homes; Group 2 = group of subjects living in
homes for the aged.

Table 4 Mutual Correlations of Level of Anxiety (LA), and Physical Self-Confidence (PhSC), Adjustment to Psychological Changes (APCh), and Prospective Feelings (PF)

Variables	1[a]	2[b]	3[b]	4
1. LA	—	−.27	−.37	.32
2. PhSC	−.26	—	.55	−.38
3. APCh	−.30	.36	—	−.36
4. PF	.40	−.20	—[c]	—

Note. All correlations significant at $p < .001$.
[a]Group 2.   [b]Group 1.   [c]Correlation coefficient has not been calculated due to insufficient value of the "hi-square" criterion.

interpreted in two ways.[5] First, low self-esteem (reflected in low PhSC and APCh scores) is assumed to be one of the major factors that induces anxiety. This assumption fits within a theoretical framework that posits that anxiety is associated with the tension that arises when there is a discrepancy between one's self-concept and the perception of reality (Rogers, 1951).

Positive correlations between self-structures and anxiety were also found in our earlier studies, conducted with Tsokov (1982). Level of self-esteem in itself was found to induce anxiety to a lesser degree than was an index based on the ratio between the image of "real self" and "ideal self." A higher level of anxiety induced by a greater discrepancy between the two substructures of the self can be accounted for by the frustration of self-needs related to an individual's inner integration.

Other investigators have also reported negative correlations between anxiety and different aspects of the self-concept. In a study of married couples, Lundgren, Jergens, and Gibson (1980) found negative correlations (−.48 for men and −.40 for women) between self-esteem and anxiety as measured by the MAS. Schafer and Keith (1981) found negative correlations between self-esteem and depression (−.40 for men and −.35 for women), the latter being deduced from the frequency of experiencing psychological distress.

Individuals who manifest a high level of anxiety, owing to higher suggestibility (Bakeev, 1971, 1974) and the disposition to interpret a wide range of events as dangerous, are likely to be more sensitive to, and to overestimate the importance of, age-induced physical and psychological changes. Positive correlations were found between these two parameters of general self-esteem that were considerably higher for subjects living in their own homes (.55) than for those living in homes for the aged (.36). There was also a prominent relation between LA and APF, indicating that high LA subjects were more likely to interpret the future in terms of uncertainty, anxiety, and danger; this correlation was higher for the subjects who lived in homes for the aged (.40 as compared with .32).

No significant relation was found between APF scores and APCh for subjects who lived in homes for the aged, and the relation between APF scores and physi-

[5]We cannot expect very high correlations among level of anxiety, self-evaluation of physical status, and adjustment to psychological changes because the modification of the 30-item Anxiety scale to measure three levels of anxiety reduced the power of the correlation coefficients. This procedure was required because, in the larger social-psychological study, it was not possible to use a wide range of scores for each item.

cal self-confidence was much weaker for this group. These findings appear to indicate that the physical and mental health of subjects who live in homes for the aged are more rarely influenced by anxiety prospective feelings (as registered by an open question) than for subjects living in their own homes. However, this interpretation was only partly confirmed by a content analysis of the responses to the open-ended question, "What causes these feelings in you?" The data obtained indicated that fear for one's health ranked third for those residing in their own homes. Adverse features of the international situation, such as fear of war and aggravation of international relations, ranked first; diffuse worries, illustrated by statements such as "fear of everything," and "uncertainty and anxiety," ranked second. It is worth noting that the fourth determinant of anxiety in the subjects who resided in their own homes was social in nature, including problems such as fear of poverty, worry about the rise in the cost of living, housing problems, inadequate pensions, depreciation of values in the young generation, and so forth.

For subjects who resided in homes for the aged, we found a tendency that was contrary to our expectations. The leading factor in the content of the anxiety prospective feeling was fear for one's health, which was ranked first by more than 40% of the subjects in this group. Fear of death ranked second and loneliness ranked third. Anxiety prospective feelings were not associated with general social problems in this group.

Clearly, our findings suggest that there was no relation between the objectively established confidence in one's physical condition and APCh to APF on the one hand, and to awareness and verbalization of the content of anxiety on the other. This raises questions about the reliability of data concerned with the determinants of emotional status of older persons that are obtained through explicit statements, for example, by means of a sociological interview. On the whole, these findings confirm the hypothesis that general self-confidence in adults, as expressed in self-evaluation of physical and psychological status and emotional attitude toward the future, is a critical psychological determinant of anxiety.

CORRELATIONS BETWEEN REALIZATION
OF LIFE PURPOSES, ANXIETY,
AND SELF-CONFIDENCE

Table 5 reports the correlations between the degree of realization of basic life purposes with LA, PhSC, APCh, and APF. For elderly people residing in their own homes, the prime determinants of anxiety seemed to be failure to attain goals connected with material welfare, education, and family and children. The most prominent correlations were between the realization of life purposes in terms of material welfare with LA and APF. Frustration of professional and social activity goals was not significantly related to level of anxiety. Unattained professional self-actualization, however, correlated with APF, although not as strongly as with unrealized material welfare goals. Most of the correlations of the realization-of-life-purposes measures with PhSC and APCh were statistically significant but relatively weaker.

The picture was somewhat different for residents of homes for the aged. There were fewer and relatively weaker correlations between the studied variables, and anxiety level for this group was not associated with unattained goals either in

Table 5 Correlations of the Degree of Realization of Life Purposes with Level of Anxiety (LA), Physical Self-Confidence (PhSC), Adjustment to Psychological Changes (APCh), and Anxiety Prospective Feeling (APF)

Field of life purposes	LA		PhSC		APCh		APF	
	1	2	1	2	1	2	1	2
Material welfare	− .40	—	.20	.18	.29	.18	− .38	− .30
Profession	—	—	.17	.19	.19	—	− .28	− .26
Family & children	− .38	− .20	—	—	—	.22	− .27	− .36
Education	− .38	—	.16	—	.30	—	− .26	—
Social activity	—	− .19	.17	.20	.20	.20	—	—

Note. All correlations significant at $p < .001$. Group 1 = subjects living in their own homes; Group 2 = subjects living in homes for the aged. Dashes indicate that the correlation coefficient has not been calculated owing to insufficient value of the "hi-square" criterion.

material welfare or in education. Strong relations were found only between APF and unattained goals in the sphere of family and children, material welfare, and profession. Logically enough, frustration of life purposes connected with family and child rearing had a stronger impact on APF for these subjects who had been torn from their home environment.

In general, the frustration of life purposes in the material welfare sphere tended to be the most important prerequisite of LA, APF, and low self-confidence. This would seem to be a natural tendency insofar as attainment of goals in the material welfare sphere forms the basis of human existence and, to a large extent, presupposes goal attainment in other spheres of life. In contrast, goals connected with social activities had the smallest impact. Frustration of life purposes in education influenced the level of anxiety and other parameters of general self-confidence only for the elderly persons living in a normal home environment.

These results lead one to touch on another question not central in the subject matter of the present study. It seems justified to conclude that the weaker correlations between anxiety and the parameters of general self-confidence with the realization of life purposes for subjects residing in homes for the aged were due to their special social status rather than to inherent personality traits. As far as level of anxiety is concerned, no statistically significant differences were found between the investigated groups, but the relative isolation from family and relatives, and the association with elderly people only, obviously reduced the impact of studied social-psychological factors of self-confidence and anxiety. The dominating content of their anxiety prospective feelings also revealed a certain withdrawal from the problems of social life.

The lack of themes connected with internal and external social problems in the subjects who were living in homes for the aged points to a predominantly egocentric orientation—fear for one's health—regardless of the fact that these individuals enjoyed free medical care at any time as well as routine medical checks. The fact that fears of death and distress because of loneliness were major themes in the content of anxiety prospective feeling also showed that the provision of food, comfortable living, and free medical care were insufficient to foster psychological well-being and cannot fully replace active social contacts.

SUMMARY AND CONCLUSIONS

The construction and development of a Bulgarian version of the Taylor (1953) MAS was described in detail. Having established that gender and age affect the reliability of some MAS items, separate but equivalent versions of the scale were developed for different age groups. The scales developed to assess trait anxiety in subjects over 50 years of age had high internal consistency reliability and were judged to be useful for measuring trait anxiety in older adults.

The present study examined the relation of trait anxiety to self-confidence and the realization of life purposes for elderly persons living in their own homes and for those residing in homes for the aged within a broad social-psychological framework. The hypothesis that high anxiety was related to low self-evaluation of physical and psychological status was generally confirmed. Level of trait anxiety was found to be related to the degree to which individuals believed they had attained basic goals in life. Frustration of life purposes in the sphere of material welfare had the greatest impact on anxiety and general self-confidence.

Qualitative differences were found in the content of the anxiety prospective feelings of persons residing in homes for the aged and those living in their own homes. Fears about health and death, and distress due to loneliness, were the predominant themes for individuals of the first group, whereas those living in their own homes reported social factors as the main determinants of their anxiety. Correlations between anxiety, self-confidence, and the realization of life purposes were also weaker for individuals living in residences for the aged as compared with subjects living at home.

REFERENCES

Bakeev, V. A. (1971). Relationship between suggestibility and anxiety. In *Proceedings of 4th Congress of the Soviet Psychological Society*. Tbilisi, USSR: Metsniereba.

Bakeev, V. A. (1974). The anxious and suggestible personality. *New Research in Psychology, 1*, 19–21.

Botwinick, J. (1973). *Aging and behavior*. New York: Springer.

Eysenck, H. J. (1970). *The structure of human personality*. London: Methuen.

Goldstein, K. (1939). *The organism: A holistic approach to biology*. New York: American Book.

Gulliksen, H. (1950). *Theory of mental tests*. New York: Wiley.

Imedadze, N. V. (1966). Anxiety as a factor of learning in preschool children. In A. S. Prangishvili (Ed.), *Psychological research* (pp. 49–57). Tbilisi, USSR: Metsniereba.

Johnson, S. C. (1967). Hierarchical clustering schemes. *Psychometrica, 32*, 241–254.

Kuhlen, R. G. (1959). Aging and life adjustment. In J. E. Birren (Ed.), *Handbook of aging and the individual* (pp. 852–900). Chicago: University of Chicago Press.

Lader, R. H. (1972). The nature of anxiety. *British Journal of Psychology, 121*, 481–491.

Levitov, N. D. (1969). The psychic condition of anxiety. *Voprosy Psychologii, 1*, 131–138.

Lundgren, D. C., Jergens, V. H., & Gibson, J. L. (1980). Marital relationships, evaluations of spouse and self, and anxiety. *Journal of Psychology, 106*, 227–240.

Mandler, G., & Watson, D. L. (1966). Anxiety and the interruption of behavior. In C. D. Spielberger (Ed.), *Anxiety and behavior* (pp. 263–288). New York: Academic Press.

May, R. (1950). *The meaning of anxiety*. New York: Ronald Press.

McDonald, R. J. (1980). *Measuring emotional status in the elderly*. Paper presented at the 22nd International Congress of Psychology, Leipzig, German Democratic Republic.

Paspalanov, I., & Stetinsky, D. (1980a). *Age dynamics and structural changes in anxiety as a personality trait*. Paper presented at the 22nd International Congress of Psychology, Leipzig, German Democratic Republic.

Paspalanov, I., & Stetinsky, D. (1980b). On the problem of level of anxiety and its measurement in psychology (II). *Psychology, 2*, 74–85.

Petrov, I. H. (1978). *Psychic and aging: Review*. Sofia, Bulgaria: Academy of Medical Sciences.

Rogers, C. R. (1951). *Client-centered therapy.* Boston: Houghton-Mifflin.

Schafer, R. B., & Keith, P. M. (1981). Self-esteem discrepancies and depression. *Journal of Psychology, 109,* 43–49.

Spielberger, C. D. (1966). Theory and research on anxiety. In C. D. Spielberger (Ed.), *Anxiety and behavior* (pp. 3–20). New York: Academic Press.

Spielberger, C. D. (1972a). Conceptual and methodological issues in anxiety research. In C. D. Spielberger (Ed.), *Anxiety: Current trends in theory and research* (Vol. 2, pp. 481–491). New York: Academic Press.

Spielberger, C. D. (1972b). Current trends in theory and research on anxiety. In C. D. Spielberger (Ed.), *Anxiety: Current trends in theory and research* (Vol. 1, pp. 3–19). New York: Academic Press.

Spielberger, C. D. (1976). The nature and measurement of anxiety. In C. D. Spielberger & R. Diaz-Guerrero (Eds.), *Cross-cultural anxiety* (Vol. 1, pp. 3–12). Washington, DC: Hemisphere/Wiley.

Stetinsky, D., & Paspalanov, I. (1980). Dynamics in a complex of symptoms of anxiety as a personality trait. In E. V. Shorochova & Z. Ivanova (Eds.), *Psychological regulation of activity* (pp. 235–266). Sofia, Bulgaria: Science and Art.

Taylor, J. A. (1953). A personality scale of manifest anxiety. *Journal of Abnormal and Social Psychology, 48,* 285–290.

Tsokov, P. G. (1982). *Relationship between level of anxiety, level of self-acceptance and personality orientation.* Unpublished master's thesis, University of Sofia, Sofia, Bulgaria.

Whitbourne, S. K. (1976). Test anxiety in elderly and young adults. *Human Development, 7,* 201–210.

APPENDIX A
Items Used in the Four Versions of the Developed Scales

	Position[a]			
	Men		Women	
Statements and key	16–30	31–50	16–30	31–50
I often doubt whether I will succeed in my work. (True)	3	3	3	3
I frequently feel uncertain. (True)	5	5	5	5
I am easily embarrassed. (True)	16	16	16	16
I am a very nervous person. (True)	18	18	18	18
I worry beyond reason all the time. (True)	23	23	23	23
Often I lose sleep over worry. (True)	25	25	25	25
I frequently notice my hand shakes when I try to do something. (True)	27	27	27	27
I often don't feel steady. (True)	29	29	29	29
I work under a great deal of strain. (True)	35	35	35	35
Often I become so excited that I find it hard to get to sleep. (True)	40	40	40	40
My sleep is restless and disturbed. (True)	49	49	49	49
I am often uncertain in my working capacity. (True)	51	51	51	51
I tend to worry about everything. (True)	53	53	53	53
Often, after an exerting exercise, I feel broken down. (True)	57	57	57	57
I am usually calm and not easily upset. (False)	60	60	60	60
Sometimes I have the feeling that I am useless. (True)	7	—	7	7
I often find myself worrying about something. (True)	9	9	—	—
My feelings are hurt easier than most people's. (True)	11	11	11	—
I have often felt that I faced so many difficulties I could not overcome them. (True)	13	—	31	31
I am not at all confident of myself. (True)	20	—	42	42
It makes me nervous to have to wait. (True)	22	22	22	—
I find it hard to keep my mind on a task or job. (True)	30	—	30	—
I am very interested and anxious to know what other people think of me. (True)	31	31	—	—
I am more self-conscious than most people. (True)	33	33	—	—
When I learn that someone has talked about me, my first thought is about something unpleasant. (True)	37	37	—	—
I often worry about failures that might happen to me. (True)	38	38	—	44
At times I think I am no good at all. (True)	42	—	33	33
I feel anxious about something or someone almost all of the time. (True)	44	44	37	—
I worry over money and business. (True)	46	46	—	—
At times I am so restless that I cannot sit in a chair for very long. (True)	47	47	—	30
I have been afraid of things or people that I know could not hurt me. (True)	—	20	20	20
I can almost always keep myself well in hand. (False)	—	—	9	9
I do not tire quickly. (False)	—	7	46	46
I am happy most of the time. (False)	—	42	—	11
Compared to my friends I am a well-balanced person. (False)	—	13	—	37
I am very confident of myself. (False)	—	—	13	13
I cry easily. (True)	—	—	47	47
I blush easily. (True)	—	30	44	—
I have very few headaches. (False)	—	—	—	22
I do not often notice my heart pounding and I am seldom short of breath. (False)	—	—	38	38

Each number indicates the position of the item in the scale. The dash indicates that this item is not included in the scale.

APPENDIX B
Distracting Questions

Position and statements

1. I enjoy the rush in work.
2. I easily switch from one activity to another.
4. I hate when I have to get up immediately after waking.
6. I have patience to explain something over and over again even when I am not understood.
8. I dislike talking with strangers in trains, buses, etc.
10. I remember faces very well.
12. I have no problems getting along with slow people.
14. Weather strongly affects my mood.
15. I prefer to stick to schedule in my everyday life.
17. I read novels quite quickly.
19. I remember better in the evening than early in the morning.
21. I enjoy housekeeping.
24. I prefer physical strain rather than mental.
26. I easily put on or take off weight.
28. I relax better among people rather than when I am alone.
32. I too often remember my childhood.
34. It is difficult for me to adjust to a new rhythm of work.
36. I prefer to take treatment by myself rather than going to a doctor.
39. I have a habit of reading while eating.
41. I enjoy reading love stories.
43. I like to be with people who don't talk too much.
45. Usually I talk quickly.
48. I can give up a discussion if I see that no one understands me.
50. In general I have no problems in communication with people.
52. I enjoy the long journeys.
54. I quickly get used to new situations.
55. I can fall asleep easily at any time.
56. Compared to other people I know I am more ready to yield.
58. I prefer work that requires movement.
59. I recover quickly from fatigue.

Note. The distracting questions have the same position in the four versions of the scale.

APPENDIX C
Level of Anxiety Scale for Men over 50

Position, statements, and key

1. I prefer physical strain rather than mental. (—)
2. I often find myself worrying about things that might happen in the future. (True)
3. I easily establish contacts with other people. (—)
4. I frequently feel uncertain. (True)
5. I have patients to explain something over and over again even when I am not understood. (—)
6. I often find myself worrying about something. (True)
7. I can almost always keep myself well in hand. (False)
8. I am happy most of the time. (False)
9. Weather strongly affects my mood. (—)
10. It makes me nervous to have to wait. (True)
11. I relax better among people rather than when I am alone. (—)
12. I am easily embarrassed. (True)
13. I am a very nervous person. (True).
14. I have been afraid of things or people that I know could not hurt me. (True).

(Table continues on next page)

APPENDIX C
Level of Anxiety Scale for Men over 50 (*Continued*)

Position, statements, and key

15. I quickly get used to new situations. (—)
16. I am more self-conscious than most people. (True)
17. I worry beyond reason all the time. (True)
18. Often I lose sleep over worry. (True)
19. I get irritated when someone talks loudly. (—)
20. I frequently notice my hand shakes when I try to do something. (True)
21. I often don't feel steady. (True)
22. At times I am so restless that I cannot sit in a chair for very long. (True)
23. I prefer walking down the streets to going out in the open air. (—)
24. I have often felt that I faced so many difficulties I could not overcome them. (True)
25. When I learn that someone has talked about me, my first thought is about something unpleasant. (True)
26. I prefer to stick to schedule in my everyday life. (—)
27. I work under a great deal of strain. (True)
28. I prefer to take treatment by myself rather than going to a doctor. (—)
29. Compared to my friends I am a well-balanced person. (False)
30. I am very interested and anxious to know what other people think of me. (True)
31. Often I become so excited that I find it hard to get to sleep. (True)
32. Compared to other people I know I am more ready to yield. (—)
33. I am not at all confident of myself. (True)
34. I worry over the health of my relatives and friends all the time. (True)
35. I do not tire quickly. (False)
36. I like to be with people that don't talk too much. (—)
37. I feel anxious about something or someone almost all of the time. (True)
38. My sleep is restless and disturbed. (True)
39. It is easier for me to remember faces than names. (—)
40. I am often uncertain in my working capacity. (True)
41. I tend to worry about everything. (True)
42. I easily come on friendly terms with children. (—)
43. Often, after an exerting exercise, I feel broken down. (True)
44. I am usually calm and not easily upset. (False)

Note. The dash indicates a distracting question.

APPENDIX D
Level of Anxiety Scale for Women over 50

Position, statements, and key

 6. Sometimes I have the feeling that I am useless. (True)
10. I am very confident of myself. (False)
16. I have very few headaches. (False)
25. At times I think I am no good at all. (True)
30. I do not often notice my heart pounding and I am seldom short of breath. (False)
37. I cry easily. (True)

Note. We list only these statements which differ from the male scale ones.

6

Personal and Interpersonal Determinants of Children's Anxiety

Yona Teichman, Miriam Ben-Rafael, and Hana Gilaie
Tel Aviv University, Israel

In the vast literature on anxiety, relatively few studies have investigated developmental and etiological issues. The research on these topics has been guided by three diverse theoretical orientations. The psychodynamic approach based on Freudian concepts claims that anxiety can be traced to the birth trauma. Later in life, anxiety is evoked when people are not able to master intense external or internal excitations, either directly or by activating appropriate defenses. These intense excitations may be caused by traumatic external situations that flood the ego with excessive stimulation, or by internal excitations resulting from intrapsychic conflicts associated with the expression of libidinal or aggressive impulses.

A second approach to explaining the origins of anxiety is based on learning principles associated with classical or vicarious conditioning. Classical conditioning theorists assume that anxiety is an innate (unconditioned) response evoked by intense noxious stimulation. When this unlearned anxiety reaction is associated with a stimulus that did not originally evoke any emotional response, the previously neutral stimulus becomes a conditioned stimulus for anxiety.

The conditioning of anxiety has been repeatedly demonstrated in numerous experiments with animals and humans. As early as 1920, Watson and Raynor demonstrated that a child, "Little Albert," with no previous fear of rats could be conditioned to fear rats and similar objects by exposing him to a sudden loud noise while he was playing with a white rat. Fears learned in the laboratory are considered by classical conditioning theorists to be analogous to phobias and neurotic anxiety (Dollard & Miller, 1950; Wolpe, 1969).

Bandura (1969, 1977) theorized that anxiety reactions are learned through a vicarious conditioning process. A basic assumption of Bandura's social learning theory is that humans acquire most of their emotional repertoire by observation rather than by experience. According to Bandura, "Vicarious emotional conditioning results from observing others experience positive or negative emotional effects in conjunction with particular stimulus events" (1969, p. 167). This implies a reciprocal dynamic interaction between a person and his environment, which Bandura (1978) labeled *reciprocal determinism*. Thus, people are influenced by their environment, but they also modify this environment and to some extent control

Miriam Ben-Rafael is now associated with the Child and Adolescent Clinic at the Geha Psychiatric Hospital, Petach-Tiqva, Israel.

their own experience and behavior. Thus, individuals are not directly driven by intrapsychic or environmental forces; rather, thoughts, feelings, and behavior result from the continuous reciprocity between internal and environmental factors.

Bandura's (1969, 1977, 1978) theory is quite similar in some respects to a third approach, which suggests that cognitive processes, rather than exposure to real or imagined dangers, precipitate anxiety. Cognitive theorists relate anxiety, as well as other emotions, to man's capability for symbolic construction. Several cognitive mechanisms that appear to activate emotional reactions have been identified. For example, Janis (1962) stressed the importance of anticipation, Lazarus (1966) emphasized cognitive appraisal, and Schachter and Singer (1962) focused on labeling environmental events on the basis of interpersonal signals. According to Janis (1971), cognitive explanations are applicable primarily to general threat cues that precede the actual danger. Averill (1976) proposed a more general cognitive explanation of the development of anxiety. According to Averill, anxiety is a state of cognitive disintegration that impairs one's ability to process information and meaningfully interpret oneself or one's environment. The causes of cognitive disintegration may be intrapsychic conflict, psychological trauma, stimulus overload or deprivation, separation from significant others, or sociocultural disorganization. Whenever the interaction between a person and his or her environment is disturbed, the potential for anxiety exists.

Empirical inquiry into the etiology of anxiety has focused primarily on learning principles and conditioning phenomena. Vicarious conditioning of fear responses has been repeatedly demonstrated with adults (Bandura & Rosenthal, 1966; Berger, 1962; Craig & Lowery, 1969; Craig & Weinstein, 1965). Research on the vicarious acquisition of emotions in children has concentrated mainly on aggressive behavior (Bandura, 1973). This is unfortunate because information obtained by studying children can contribute to understanding developmental and etiological issues.

Two studies that investigated the vicarious acquisition of emotions in children are briefly mentioned. Venn and Short (1973) demonstrated the vicarious conditioning of negative and positive emotions in nursery school children who watched a film in which a peer model manifested either fear responses (screaming, withdrawing) or positive emotions (smiling, approaching). The results indicated that vicarious experience influenced the observer's reaction to a neutral stimulus paired with the model's response. However, the effects were relatively temporary and could be neutralized by instructions, reinforcement conditions, or both. Similarly, Morris, Brown, and Halbert (1977) reported that anxiety increased in nursery school children who observed an anxious peer model and decreased after the children viewed a nonanxious model. Although these studies demonstrated that vicarious learning was involved in the acquisition of anxiety, only the environmental influence was examined. The personal determinants that might influence anxiety were not evaluated.

In Spielberger's (1966, 1972) trait–state theory of anxiety, the critical personality variable involved in determining an individual's experience of anxiety is anxiety proneness, that is, individual differences in the disposition to experience anxiety. Spielberger differentiated between two anxiety constructs: transitory or state anxiety (A-State) and anxiety proneness as a personality trait (A-Trait). The trait–state anxiety theory hypothesizes that persons high in A-Trait are more prone to experience elevations in A-State in stressful interpersonal situations. To measure the two aspects of anxiety in adolescents and adults, Spielberger, Gorsuch, and Lushene (1970) developed the State–Trait Anxiety Inventory (STAI). The State–Trait Anxiety Inventory for Children (STAIC) was constructed to assess anxiety in 8- to 12-year-olds (Spielberger, Edwards, Lushene, Montuori, & Platzek, 1973).

The STAI and the STAIC were translated and adapted into Hebrew by Teichman and Melnick (1979). In the two studies that are reported in this chapter, the Hebrew adaptations of the STAI and the STAIC were used to evaluate relations between the trait anxiety of children and their reactions to anxiety-relevant cues in adults with whom they interacted. To be more specific, the influence of situational factors and individual differences in trait anxiety on the vicarious acquisition of state anxiety in child–adult interactions was investigated. Concentration on child–adult interactions seemed especially appropriate because of the long exposure of children to adults during a period of high vulnerability and dependency.

The investigation of the influence of an adult model on a child's experience of anxiety (A-State) expands on the findings reported in previous studies (Morris et al., 1977; Venn & Short, 1973) in which the environmental influence of peers on children's emotional reactions was demonstrated. This general approach is also consistent with Bandura's (1978) theory on person–environment reciprocity and the views of most cognitive theorists (Averill, 1976; Schachter, 1964; Schachter & Singer, 1962). The following hypotheses were evaluated: (a) High A-Trait children experience higher A-State than do low A-Trait children in most situations, (b) children exposed to anxious adults experience higher A-State, and (c) high A-Trait children who observe anxious adults experience a greater increase in A-State than do low A-Trait children. These hypotheses were tested in two studies.

STUDY 1: EFFECTS OF A-TRAIT
AND OBSERVATION OF AN ANXIOUS MODEL
ON A-STATE

The first study was conducted in a laboratory setting. Before the experiment, the STAIC was administered to 64 eleven- to 12-year-old girls in a neutral classroom situation. The children were then divided into high and low trait-anxiety groups, which were defined on the basis of STAIC scores. Baseline state anxiety was determined, and half of each group was exposed to a film presentation of an anxious model performing a task; the other half watched a calm model performing the same task.

The model in both films was a blindfolded young woman stacking 20 blocks with her nonpreferred hand. The procedure was adapted from one described by Perry and Millimet (1977). The performance sequence and achievement on the task were the same in both films. The anxious model manifested behaviors such as hair pulling, lip chewing, and excessive restlessness that distracted her from the task; the calm model exhibited relaxed behavior. After viewing the film, the child's level of A-State was again assessed with the STAIC. The child was then asked to perform the same task that was demonstrated by the model.

The first question addressed in this study was whether exposure to the anxious or calm model had different effects on children's A-State. Both children with high and children with low trait anxiety who were exposed to the anxious model experienced a significant increase in A-State ($p < .05$); the anxiety level of children exposed to the calm model did not show a significant change. Thus, exposing children to an anxious adult significantly increased the child's level of A-State intensity.

Did children who were high or low in trait anxiety react differently? Did the model's anxiety differentially affect children who differed in trait anxiety? To answer these questions, a 2 × 2 between-groups analysis of variance (ANOVA) was performed in which the independent variables were the child's trait anxiety (high vs. low) and the behavior of the model (anxious vs. calm). The dependent variable was the level of A-State experienced by each child immediately after viewing the film, but before performing on the task. The mean A-State scores of the high and low A-Trait children who observed the anxious and calm models are presented in Figure 1. Both main effects were statistically significant. The high A-Trait children manifested higher levels of state anxiety in both situations, $F(2, 59) = 7.38$, $p < .01$; children exposed to the anxious model showed higher levels of A-State than did those exposed to the calm model, $F(2, 59) = 6.47$, $p < .01$. The interaction effect was not significant.

STUDY 2: EFFECTS OF PARENTAL ANXIETY ON CHILDREN HIGH OR LOW IN A-TRAIT

This study examined the same hypotheses tested in the previous study in a significant real-life interpersonal interaction. The subjects were 60 six- to twelve-

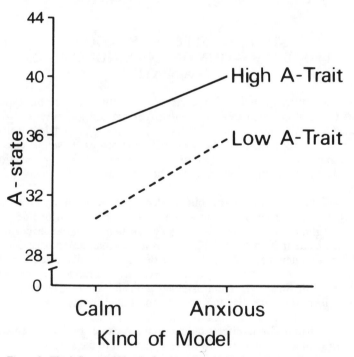

Figure 1 The influence of level of trait anxiety (A-Trait) and kind of model on the subjects' state-anxiety (A-State) level.

Table 1   Means, Standard Deviations and t Values of Parents' A-State and A-Trait in the Two Hospitalization Settings

Anxiety	t	Hospital	Day clinic
A-Trait	2.45**		
M		33.30	39.79
SD		7.60	12.23
n		30	28
A-State	1.35*		
M		41.52	45.60
SD		14.30	12.00
n		30	29

*$p < .10$.   **$p < .01$.

year-old hospitalized children (27 boys and 33 girls) and their parents (44 mothers and 16 fathers) drawn from the pediatric facilities of two major Israeli hospitals (Sheba and Belinson). Thirty children and the parent who accompanied each child were studied in both settings. In both hospitals, the main diagnoses at admission were comparable and the length of stay was 3–5 days. The children at Sheba were hospitalized in an ordinary ward; the children at Belinson were examined and treated in a day clinic program. They returned home each day in the afternoon or evening. There were no demographic differences between the samples, which were matched on the hospitalized child's age, sex, number of siblings, and country of origin and the parents' educational level.

The parents' anxiety level was defined in terms of the amount of anxiety attributed to them by their children. To compare the findings of the two studies, this perceived parental anxiety was assessed by asking the children to indicate their parent's feelings by responding to the Hebrew STAIC, which was also used to assess the child's own feelings. The children rated their parent's anxiety by completing the STAIC A-State Scale with directions to report their parent's feelings at the moment. A pilot study with a comparable sample of healthy children, in which the anxiety of the parents was evaluated with the Hebrew STAI, indicated that children are reasonably accurate in evaluating their parents' anxiety. The correlation in the pilot study between the anxiety reported by parents and that perceived by their healthy children was .67. This correlation in the present study was .49.

Differences in the mean A-Trait and A-State scores, and in perceived parental anxiety for children in the two hospital settings, were evaluated with t tests; no significant differences were found. However, the actual A-Trait and A-State scores of the parents of children treated in the day clinic were significantly higher than those of the parents of the children hospitalized on the regular wards. The means, standard deviations, and t values for these comparisons are presented in Table 1.

Within each hospital sample, the children were divided into four subgroups on the basis of their A-Trait scores (high vs. low) and the anxiety attributed to their parents (high vs. low). The effect of each child's trait anxiety and perceived parental anxiety on the child's state anxiety was evaluated in 2×2 between-groups ANOVAs performed separately for each hospital setting. The mean A-State scores for the four groups of children in the ordinary hospital setting are plotted in Figure 2, in which it may be noted that the pattern of means was very similar to those obtained in the laboratory experiment with the anxious and calm models (see

Figure 1). As in Study 1, the main effects for trait anxiety, $F(2, 29) = 6.23, p < .01$, and perceived parental anxiety, $F(2, 29) = 13.03, p < .01$, were both significant, but the interaction effect was not.

The pattern of anxiety means for the children hospitalized in the day clinic was quite different. In addition to the main effects of children's A-Trait, $F(2, 29) = 4.03, p < .05$, and perceived parental anxiety, $F(2, 29) = 18.93, p < .01$, the interaction between these variables was significant, $F(2, 29) = 12.72, p < .01$. The mean A-State scores of the low and the high A-Trait children who attributed high or low anxiety to their parents are reported in Figure 3. Although the mean A-State scores of the low A-Trait children were similar to those found for the low A-Trait children hospitalized on regular wards and in the laboratory study, the high A-Trait children were more strongly influenced by their environment. When they perceived their parents as calm, they were very calm; however, when they perceived their parents as anxious, their A-State level was sharply elevated.

DISCUSSION OF THE FINDINGS
AND THEIR THEORETICAL IMPLICATIONS

In both studies, anxiety predisposition (A-Trait) and interpersonal environmental variables (i.e., anxious model or parent) influenced the children's state anxiety reactions. However, a significant interaction between these factors was found only

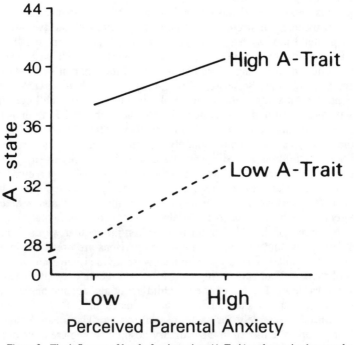

Figure 2 The influence of level of trait anxiety (A-Trait) and perceived parental anxiety on subjects' state-anxiety (A-State) level in the hospital.

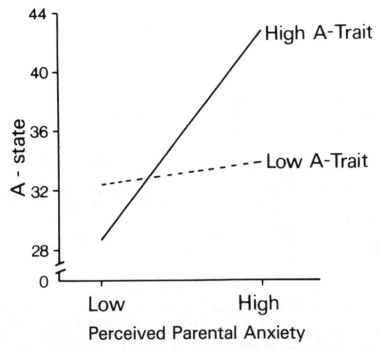

Figure 3 The influence of levels of trait anxiety (A-Trait) and perceived parental anxiety on subjects' state-anxiety (A-State) level in the day clinic.

for the children hospitalized in the day clinic. These findings are consistent with theories that emphasize the influence of both person and environment in evoking emotional reactions (Averill, 1976; Bandura, 1969, 1977; Schacter, 1964; Schacter & Singer, 1962). The results also support the social learning theory position that emotional reactions, as well as many other behaviors, can be acquired by observational learning (i.e., by vicarious conditioning).

The findings also support Spielberger's (1966, 1972) trait–state anxiety theory—in particular, the relation predicted between state and trait anxiety. According to Spielberger, persons high in trait anxiety tend to react with higher levels of state anxiety in emotionally arousing situations. Although this pattern has been demonstrated repeatedly in studies with adults (Auerbach, 1973; Lamb, 1973; Spielberger, Auerbach, Wadsworth, Dunn, & Taulbee, 1973), it was replicated in the present study in school-aged children; those with higher trait anxiety were consistently higher in state anxiety (see Figures 1 and 2). In the day clinic setting, which had the highest potential for anxiety-arousing cues, the high A-Trait children who perceived their parents as anxious showed the most elevated state-anxiety reaction.

The finding that high A-Trait children in the day clinic who perceived their parents as less anxious manifested the lowest level of state anxiety (see Figure 3) seems to contradict Spielberger's theory; on further consideration, however, this finding can be explained within the context of trait–state anxiety theory. According to Spielberger (1966, 1972), high A-Trait scores reflect an individual's disposition to respond with higher A-State in interpersonal situations perceived as threats to self-esteem, that is, ego threats. In the hospital settings of the present study, the parents who added anxiety cues greatly increased the state-anxiety level of their high A-Trait children, whereas the parents who were calm appeared to reduce the state anxiety of such children, supporting Spielberger's theory that high A-Trait individuals are especially sensitive to anxiety cues in significant interpersonal relationships such as parent–child interactions.

The findings of the research reported in this chapter provide strong evidence that the state–trait relation is influenced by social and environmental factors. Irrespective of their level of trait anxiety, the children who observed anxious adults reacted with higher levels of A-State than did those exposed to less-anxious adults, as can be noted in Figures 1 and 2. The significant interaction between the personality and environmental variables, which emerged only in the day clinic setting (see Figure 3), was found in the situation that was most threatening for the parents. Although the difference between the state-anxiety means of the two groups of parents (see Table 1) only approached statistical significance ($p < .10$), the A-State means for both groups were very high, suggesting that a ceiling effect may have reduced this difference.

Day clinics, which are generally assumed to be less threatening for children who need medical care, are apparently highly threatening for some parents. This may be attributed to the fact that in day clinics, parents feel greater responsibility for their child's well-being than do parents whose children are hospitalized in a regular hospital. Unfortunately, because of differences in the trait-anxiety level of the two groups of parents in Study 2, it was not possible to determine whether the higher A-State scores of the day clinic parents were due to their higher level of trait anxiety or to their reactions to the hospital setting. Clearly, the influence of the two kinds of hospital settings on the anxiety reactions of parents and children merits further empirical investigations.

In the studies reported in this chapter, the influence of the emotions of adults on the emotional experiences of children exposed to them was examined. As expected, the adults perceived as experiencing a high level of emotional arousal transmitted their anxiety to children, particularly to the children high in trait anxiety. However, there are situations in which high A-Trait children who perceive their parents as calm not only tolerate the stress, but experience even lower state anxiety than do low A-Trait children (see Figure 3). It is interesting to note that the low A-Trait children in both studies reacted in an almost identical manner. When exposed to anxious adults, the state anxiety of these children increased. However, they were less sensitive to the anxiety of the adults and reported lower levels of state anxiety than did children with high trait anxiety.

On the basis of the findings reported in this chapter, it may be concluded that state anxiety in children is determined by both personality dispositions and interpersonal, anxiety-related cues. The manner in which these personality and environmental variables influence the A-State reactions of children seems to depend on the level of environmental stress. When the stress level is low, both variables contribute independently to the emotional state of the child. When emotional arousal is high, these variables interact in such a way that the environmental variables have greater influence on children with a high predisposition to anxiety. The findings indicate that theories about the etiology of anxiety must consider both individual differences in personality and anxiety-arousing environmental factors, as well as interactions among them in different kinds of situations. Neither internally oriented psychodynamic theories nor externally oriented theories such as classical conditioning can account for all of the determinants that appear to be involved in evoking anxiety reactions. Cognitive and social learning theories seem to provide a broader conceptual framework for understanding the mechanisms that evoke anxiety.

Following Bandura's (1978) concept of reciprocal determination, it would seem important to investigate not only the interactions among personality and environmental variables, but also the reciprocal intervening processes. In what way do adults with various personality characteristics influence different kinds of children in various situations, and what kinds of mutual feedback are generated by this interactive process? Although such questions are difficult to investigate, the findings reported in this chapter strongly indicate that the emotional states of adults have a significant impact on the anxiety reactions of children who are exposed to or interact with them. Because children react to the emotional cues transmitted by adults, especially in threatening situations, from a practical point of view it is essential for clinicians who work with children to take into account the variables that influence anxiety in adults. By reducing parental anxiety, children's experiences of anxiety can be indirectly influenced.

SUMMARY

The effects of personality and environmental influences on state anxiety were examined in two studies. In the first study, children with high or low trait anxiety were exposed to films presenting anxious and calm models performing a task. The children's state anxiety was influenced by both the behavior of the model and the child's predisposition to experience anxiety. In the second study, the state-anxiety level of hospitalized children with high or low trait anxiety was influenced by their own trait-anxiety level and by the perceived level of their parent's anxiety. When the emotional arousal of the parent was very high, children with high trait anxiety manifested greater sensitivity to parental cues than did low trait-anxiety children. The findings in both studies support Spielberger's (1966, 1972) theory that anxiety states are determined by the individual's disposition to experience anxiety and by social-interpersonal factors.

The results were discussed from theoretical and practical points of view. It was suggested that cognitive and social learning theories that encompass both personality and environmental factors provide the best conceptual framework for understanding the etiology of anxiety reactions and the mediating mechanisms that evoke anxiety. Because children react to emotional cues transmitted by adults, from a practical point of view it was suggested that the conditions that influence the anxiety of significant adults be taken into account as a means for indirectly controlling the anxiety of children.

REFERENCES

Auerbach, S. M. (1973). Emotional reaction to surgery. *Journal of Consulting and Clinical Psychology, 40,* 264–271.

Averill, J. R. (1976). Emotion and anxiety. Sociocultural, biological and psychological determinants. In

M. Zuckerman & C. D. Spielberger (Eds.), *Emotion and anxiety. New concepts, methods and applications* (pp. 87–130). Hillsdale, NJ: Erlbaum.

Bandura, A. (1969). *Principles of behavior modification.* New York: Holt, Rinehart & Winston.

Bandura, A. (1973). *A social-learning analysis.* Englewood Cliffs, NJ: Prentice-Hall.

Bandura, A. (1977). *Social learning theory.* Engelwood Cliffs, NJ: Prentice-Hall.

Bandura, A. (1978). The self system in reciprocal determinism. *American Psychologist, 33,* 344–358.

Bandura, A. L., & Rosenthal, T. L. (1966). Vicarious classical conditioning as a function of arousal level. *Journal of Personality and Social Psychology, 3,* 54–62.

Berger, S. M. (1962). Conditioning through vicarious instigation. *Psychological Review, 69,* 450–466.

Craig, K. D., & Lowery, H. J. (1969). Heart-rate components of conditioned vicarious automatic responses. *Journal of Personality and Social Psychology, 11,* 381–387.

Craig, K. D., & Weinstein, M. S. (1965). Conditioning vicarious affective arousal. *Psychological Reports, 17,* 955–963.

Dollard, J., & Miller, N. E. (1950). *Personality and psychotherapy: An analysis in terms of learning, thinking and culture.* New York: McGraw-Hill.

Janis, I. L. (1962). Psychological effects of warning. In G. W. Baker & D. W. Chapman (Eds.), *Man and society in disaster* (pp. 55–92). New York: Basic Books.

Janis, I. L. (1971). *Stress and frustration.* New York: Harcourt Brace Jovanovich.

Lamb, D. H. (1973). The effects of two stressors on state anxiety for students who differ in trait anxiety. *Journal of Research in Personality, 7,* 116–126.

Lazarus, R. S. (1966). *Psychological stress and the coping process.* New York: McGraw-Hill.

Morris, L. W., Brown, N. R., & Halbert, B. L. (1977). Effects of symbolic modeling on the arousal of cognitive and effective components of anxiety in pre-school children. In C. D. Spielberger & I. G. Sarason (Eds.), *Stress and anxiety* (Vol. 4, pp. 153–170). New York: Wiley.

Perry, N. W., & Millimet, C. R. (1977). Child rearing antecedents of low and high anxiety eighth grade children. In C. D. Spielberger & I. G. Sarason (Eds.), *Stress and anxiety* (Vol. 4, pp. 189–204). New York: Wiley.

Schacter, S. S. (1964). The interaction of cognitive and physiological determinants of emotional state. In L. Berkowitz (Ed.), *Advances in experimental social psychology* (Vol. 1, pp. 49–81). New York: Academic Press.

Schacter, S. S., & Singer, J. E. (1962). Cognitive, social and physiological determinants of emotional state. *Psychological Review, 69,* 379–399.

Spielberger, C. D. (1966). Theory and research on anxiety. In C. D. Spielberger (Ed.), *Anxiety and behavior* (pp. 3–20). New York: Academic Press.

Spielberger, C. D. (1972). Conceptual and methodological issues in anxiety research. In C. D. Spielberger (Ed.), *Anxiety: Current trends in theory and research* (Vol. 2, pp. 481–493). New York: Academic Press.

Spielberger, C. D., Auerbach, S. M., Wadsworth, A. P., Dunn, T. M., & Taulbee, E. S. (1973). Emotional reaction to surgery. *Journal of Consulting and Clinical Psychology, 40,* 33–38.

Spielberger, C. D., Edwards, C. D., Lushene, R. E., Montuori, J., & Platzek, D. (1973). *Preliminary test manual for the State-Trait Anxiety Inventory for Children.* Palo Alto, CA: Consulting Psychologists Press.

Spielberger, C. D., Gorsuch, R. L., & Lushene, R. E. (1970). *Manual for the State-Trait Anxiety Inventory (self-evaluation questionnaire).* Palo Alto, CA: Consulting Psychologists Press.

Teichman, Y., & Melnick, C. (1979). *The Hebrew Manual for the State-Trait Anxiety Inventory.* Tel Aviv, Israel: Tel Aviv University.

Venn, J. R., & Short, J. G. (1973). Vicarious classical conditioning of emotional responses in nursery school children. *Journal of Personality and Social Psychology, 28,* 249–255.

Watson, J. B., & Raynor, R. (1920). Conditioned emotional responses. *Journal of Experimental Psychology, 3,* 1–14.

Wolpe, J. (1969). *The practice of behavior therapy.* New York: Pergamon Press.

II

ANXIETY, COPING, AND PERFORMANCE

7

Anxious-Defensive, Anxious-Sensitive, and Nonanxious Coping Styles in Achievement-Related Stress Situations

Rainer Wieland-Eckelman
Bergische Universität-Gesamthochschule,
Federal Republic of Germany

Current criticism of theoretical conceptualizations of achievement-related anxiety research has focused on the following four issues. First, it has been argued that the performance-debilitating effect of anxiety becomes problematic when real-life situations are investigated rather than artificial laboratory tasks (see Krohne & Rogner, 1982; Krohne & Schaffner, 1980; Laux & Vossel, 1982). Second, although the influence of anxiety on achievement has been extensively investigated, little attention has been given to antecedent factors such as the opportunity to prepare and the length of preparation time (Krohne & Rogner, 1982). Third, investigators have not distinguished between the coping strategies that are used before the performance situation and the coping activities that are used during achievement-related tasks (see Krohne & Rogner, 1982). Finally, most studies to date have failed to investigate the influence of objective or perceived "degrees of freedom" with respect to goal setting, decision making, and the organization of work and recovery periods (i.e., the sequence and time structure of actions; Wieland, 1981).

The research described in this chapter endeavors to overcome some of these limitations in achievement-related anxiety research. In the first section of the chapter, the experimental paradigm and methodology that was used in a study examining individual coping styles in achievement-related stress situations are described. In the second section, the impact on task performance of anxious-defensive, anxious-sensitive, and nonanxious coping styles is discussed in the context of a detailed analysis of the microstructure of actions. The results of an investigation of the relation between anxiety-related coping activities and the macrostructure of actions are presented in the final section.

The research reported in this chapter was supported by a grant from Bundesministerium des Inneren der Bundesrepublik Deutschland (Umweltbundesamt) to Professor W. Schönpflug.

I am grateful to Professor Bösel, Professor Schönpflug, and especially to Dr. Reisenzein for their comments on an earlier version of this chapter.

INDIVIDUAL COPING STYLES
IN AN ACHIEVEMENT-RELATED
STRESSFUL SITUATION

This investigation was guided by the theoretical framework of our research group at the Free University of Berlin (see Schönpflug & Battman, 1982; Schönpflug & Wieland, 1982). It began with a detailed analysis of a real-life workplace (clerical work). On the basis of individual interviews in the work setting, experimental tasks and conditions similar to the selected workplace were constructed. The subjects' degrees of freedom with respect to individual goal setting, decision making, and the organization of work and recovery periods were incorporated in the tasks to be solved, which varied in difficultly and content. Corresponding to the increasing use of computer technology in administrative work, the subjects used a video screen and a keyboard with computer-assisted instructions in performing their tasks.

By pressing different keys, the subject could request all kinds of information that was relevant for task solution (see Figure 1). Each task consisted of a single problem with four or five alternative decisions, of which one was considered optimal. By pressing a key, the subject could request 1–12 pieces of information (e.g., price lists, specified orders, personnel data, etc.) that were needed to solve the task. Depending on the nature of the task (e.g., checking bills, controlling checks), up to 6 pieces of information were required for task solution. A directory, or survey list, containing the name of each item and the number of an associated key to be pressed to obtain information on that item was also displayed on the screen.

To illustrate the nature of one of the experimental tasks (e.g., "checking bills"), the directory read, "list of orders—press key one," "price-lists—press key two," and so forth. Although the text describing the problem always remained on the left part of the screen, the directory or the single information items could only be requested alternatively. No restrictions were imposed concerning the frequency or sequence of requests for the directory, the individual pieces of information, or the list of available decision alternatives.

The subjects were required to solve eight blocks of problems, each consisting of 8–15 subproblems. The first four blocks consisted of 10 successive tasks, all with a similar structure (checking bills, calculating bills, filling out application forms, controlling checks). Consequently, the same directory could be used for these four blocks of problems. In addition, there were three blocks of 8 successive problems, consisting of mixed tasks such as tax declarations, applications for welfare, or rent rebates. Each of these tasks consisted of the following 3 subtasks: First, checking a list of 100 lines and searching for one relevant piece of information out of this list; second, working on the main task problem; and finally, checking the correctness of the chosen decision alternative by means of mathematical calculations. In addition, requests for information on these mixed tasks were also more restricted. That is, except for the five pieces of information (three relevant and two irrelevant for reaching the optimal solution in the main task) that could be requested in any order whatsoever, all other information had to be requested in these blocks in a fixed order.

Finally, the eighth block of problems, containing 15 successive tasks, required checking operations only. More specifically, out of a list of 100 lines certain pieces

KEYBOARD

SL	DA	PT	CL	C	P
		TP			

7	8	9	E1
4	5	6	E2
1	2	3	E3
0	E4	E5	

SL = SURVEY LIST
DA = DECISION ALTERNATIVES
TP = TEXT OF THE PROBLEM
PT = PROOF-TASK
CL = CHECK LIST
C = KEY FOR PAGING
     THE SCREEN
P = KEY FOR DECLARING
     A REST-PAUSE

E1 - E5 = DECISIONS
0 - 9 = PIECES OF
         INFORMATION

Figure 1 Keyboard; respectively, keys for requesting the kinds of information relevant for task solution.

of information (e.g., personnel data such as age, monthly wages, or kinds of jobs) had to be detected. Finally, in all tasks the number of detected, relevant data had to be fed into the keyboard.

Subjects

The subjects were unemployed clerical workers from a local labor office. Seventy-two persons (50% of whom were women) participated in the investigation. They were given the equivalent of about $3.50 per hr plus some extra gratification if they had solved a minimum number of problems correctly within a certain time limit.

Procedure

The subjects were tested individually in a session lasting about 1½ days. On the first day, they were asked to first complete various questionnaires (for detailed information, see Schönpflug & Wieland, 1982; Wieland, 1984). Subsequently, to familiarize the subjects with the screen, the keyboard, and the different kinds of tasks that had to be solved in the testing situation, subjects were asked to work on a computer-assisted training program. Subjects could work through the training program as often as they wanted to, and there were no time limits imposed.

On the second day, subjects were extensively informed about the nature of the test program (i.e., the kind of tasks that had to be solved, the available options, and the working conditions) and were then asked to begin working on the tasks. The test program was divided into three phases: First, five blocks of tasks had to be completed, then there was a 15-min rest pause, and subsequently the subjects had to work on the last three blocks of tasks.

Dependent Variables

Self-Report Data

State anxiety was assessed at three stages of the performance situation (using the State–Trait Anxiety Inventory, or STAI; German version by Laux, Glanzmann, Schaffner, & Spielberger, 1981): the anticipation stage (before the computer-assisted training program [State 1]), the confrontation stage (immediately before the subjects were given the test program instructions [State 2]), and finally, the evaluation stage (immediately after the testing [State 3]. See Figure 2.)

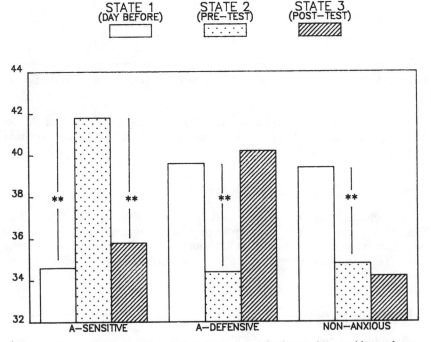

Figure 2 Temporal patterns of state anxiety for anxious-defensive, anxious-sensitive, and non-anxious subjects.

Additionally, at the end of each block of tasks, self-reported general activation and emotional well-being were measured. Furthermore, self-report data concerning performance attributions and perceived task demands, as well the perceived efficiency of individual coping strategies, were assessed.

Objective Performance Indices

Corresponding to the operations necessary to solve the different kind of tasks, the following performance indices were calculated: (a) time spent on problem identification, (b) time spent on relevant pieces of information, (c) frequency of requests for relevant pieces of information, (d) frequency of requests for directories and decision alternatives, (e) performance outcome (defined as the number of correct solutions), (f) time-related efficiency (defined as the ratio between the number of correct solutions and the time spent on task execution), and (g) action-related efficiency (defined as the ratio between the number of correct solutions and the number of operations performed).

On the basis of prior research, the task demands imposed on the subjects, as well as empirical findings from previous investigations (see Schulz & Battmann, 1980; Schulz & Schönpflug, 1982; Schönpflug & Schulz, 1979), made classifications of blocks of tasks according to their difficulty plausible.

Classification of Subjects

Because recent research on the sensitization-repression concept (see Asendorpf, Walbott, & Scherer, 1983; Krohne & Rogner, 1982; Krohne & Schaffner, 1980; Weinberger, Schwartz, & Davidson, 1979) suggests a distinction among three different habitual anxiety-related coping styles, which could be labeled *anxious-defensive, anxious-sensitive,* and *nonanxious,* we attempted to classify our subjects into three corresponding groups before the main data analysis. This was done by considering (a) the level of anxiety at the first measurement point (i.e., the day before the actual testing situation) and (b) the pretest and posttest anxiety change scores. The temporal pattern of anxiety considered characteristic of the three groups is shown in Figure 2. We assumed that anxious-sensitive and nonanxious subjects, respectively, represent those being classified as high anxious and low anxious in the trait–state model (see Spielberger, 1972, 1975), whereas anxious-defensive subjects represent those classified by Weinberger et al. (1979) and Asendorpf et al. (1983) as repressors, that is, subjects who use a repressive style of coping with achievement-related anxiety.

It might be mentioned that additional analyses suggested that these three groups also differ with regard to acquired coping modes (e.g., shifts in aspiration level when confronted with different kinds of stressful events, as well as with regard to the attributions they gave for their performance; see Weiner, 1982). It was found that anxious-defensive subjects ($n = 23$) attributed their failures more frequently to internal, unstable causes (i.e., conscious attention and self-imposed time pressure) than did anxious-sensitive ($n = 17$) and nonanxious subjects ($n = 32$). For more information on the theoretical considerations underlying this classification of subjects, see Wieland (1984).

RESULTS

The analysis and interpretation of the data presented in the following paragraphs was guided (a) by Eysenck's (1982) suggestion that although anxious individuals under certain circumstances (e.g., good preparation conditions or easy tasks) could achieve the same performance level as nonanxious subjects, their efficiency could be inferior as they invest a greater amount of effort, and (b) by Wieland's (1984) findings that nonanxious, anxious-sensitive, and anxious-defensive subjects (as defined by differing temporal patterns of state anxiety, see preceding section) do indeed use quite different, definable habitual problem- and emotion-focused styles of coping in achievement-related stress situations.

Temporal Patterns of State Anxiety and the Microstructure of Actions

According to the tasks that had to be solved in the test program (see Procedure section), the cognitive requirements imposed on the subjects and the operations necessary to solve the different tasks can be summarized as follows: (a) problem identification, (b) goal setting, (c) information seeking, (d) checking information, (e) information processing, (f) decision making, and (g) evaluation of results. The duration, number, and sequence of the orientation and control operations mentioned earlier (see Hacker, 1982; Schönpflug, 1983) are termed the *microstructure* of actions (see Schönpflug & Wieland, 1982; Wieland, 1981).

Performance Outcome, Efficiency, and Task Difficulty

Eysenck's (1982) hypothesis that anxious individuals under certain circumstances could achieve the same performance level as nonanxious individuals was supported by the finding that anxious-sensitive subjects reached the same performance level as nonanxious subjects and had lower scores regarding the time-related efficiency than did nonanxious subjects, $F(2, 69) = 8.01$, $p < .001$. Anxious-defensive persons also had significantly lower time-related efficiency scores. Their performance level, however, was significantly lower than that of nonanxious and anxious-sensitive subjects, $F(2, 69) = 5.86$, $p < .0$ (see Figure 3). This latter finding may be explained if one considers the efficiency scores for easy, medium, and difficult tasks separately.

As is demonstrated in Figure 4, the differences in time-related efficiency presented in Figure 3 are due primarily to the difficult tasks, at least if one compares anxious-sensitive and nonanxious subjects; these groups do not differ significantly with respect to medium and easy tasks. In contrast, the anxious-defensive group has significantly lower scores than the other groups in tasks of medium difficulty and is even inferior with respect to easy tasks.

Interestingly, we found similar differences among the three groups with respect to a subjective measure of efficiency. This subjective measure was obtained by computing the ratio between subjective estimates of task difficulty and performance level achieved (at the end of each block of tasks, subjects were given feedback about their achievement level). Anxious-defensive subjects tended to score significantly lower on this efficiency index than did the other two groups (anxious-defensive group—$M = 26.28$, $SD = 6.56$; anxious-sensitive group—$M = 35.05$, $SD = 7.23$; nonanxious group—$M = 34.20$, $SD = 6.98$),

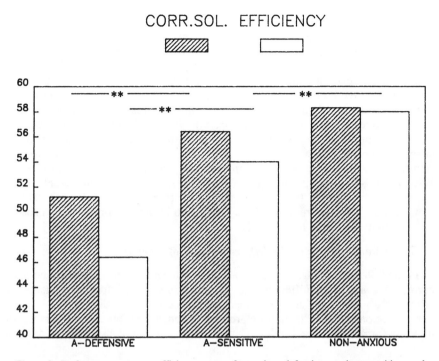

Figure 3 Performance outcome efficiency scores for anxious-defensive, anxious-sensitive, and nonanxious subjects.

$F(2, 69) = 2.76, p < .07$. In contrast to time-related efficiency, there were no significant differences between the groups with respect to action-related efficiency (ratio between number of correct solutions and number of operations performed) for medium and difficult tasks (see Figure 5). Provided that the time-related efficiency index primarily represents the quality or speed of information processing and the action-related efficiency index reflects the quality of strategy-formation processes, it seems reasonable to assume that anxious-defensive subjects had developed action strategies that were as efficient as those of the other groups.

Further support for this assumption is gained if one considers merely the number of operations performed. There were no differences among the groups with respect to the frequency of the different operations executed for solving the different blocks of tasks. This result fits well with prior data concerning individual coping modes (see Wieland, 1984), which demonstrate that there were no differences between anxious-sensitive, anxious-defensive, and nonanxious subjects with respect to their stated "disposition to change action strategies under stress."

On the other hand, the assumptions for easy tasks were not supported (see Figure 5). Nonanxious subjects had lower, and anxious-defensive subjects had significantly lower, action-related efficiency scores ($p < .01$) than did anxious-sensitive subjects. Assuming that anxious-sensitive subjects represent largely those being described as high anxious in the trait–state model, this finding constitutes additional empirical evidence for Eysenck's (1982) hypothesis that, given easy tasks, anxious subjects perform as well or even better than do nonanxious subjects.

In sum, on the basis of the data reported in this section, it may be concluded

that the anxious-defensive coping style is associated (a) with impairments of information processing or limitations of working memory, and (b) with the inability to
allocate available resources to task requirements (e.g., Eysenck, 1982; Kahneman,
1973; Pribram & McGuinness, 1975; Sanders, 1983).

Further evidence for this conclusion was obtained from the following result.
Anxious-sensitive and nonanxious subjects had a strong positive correlation between psychometrically assessed intelligence and time-related efficiency (rs = .48
and .52, respectively; p < .01 in both cases), whereas the corresponding correlation for the anxious-defensive group was near zero. Comparable results were obtained with respect to action-related efficiency. Considering that there were no
significant differences among the three groups with respect to intelligence (see
Wieland, 1984) and with respect to the standard deviations of the efficiency
scores, this result may be taken to suggest that for anxious-defensive subjects
motivational factors were more closely related to information-processing capacity
than to ability (see also Janis, 1982).

Correlation Analysis of the Different Kinds of Operations

In the following paragraph, the analysis is extended to an analysis of the intercorrelations among the different kinds of operations (e.g., information intake and
information processing) and performance outcome (see preceding section).

As mentioned earlier, the testing problem included three blocks of tasks that had
to be performed in a fixed order. That is, in these three blocks of tasks only the

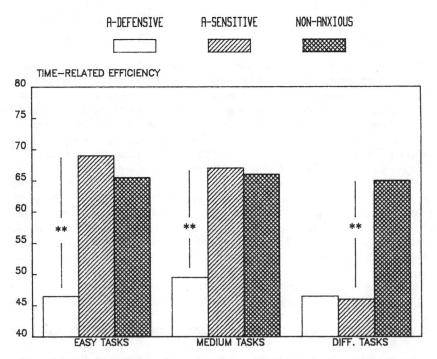

Figure 4 Time-related efficiency for easy, medium, and difficult tasks for anxious-defensive,
anxious-sensitive, and nonanxious subjects.

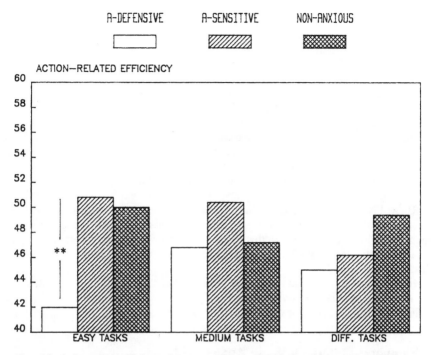

Figure 5   Action-related efficiency for easy, medium, and difficult tasks for anxious-defensive, anxious-sensitive, and nonanxious subjects.

five pieces of information (three relevant and two irrelevant for optimal solution) could be requested in any order whatsoever; all other information had to be requested in a fixed order. Because most subjects requested even these five pieces of information in the same order, it was possible to interpret any differences between the intercorrelation matrixes of the three groups as being due to differences in information processing; as there was no confounding with time and sequence, the different kind of information was processed.

The first result of interest in this context is the correlation between number of correct solutions (CS) and time spent on relevant pieces of information (TRI; see Table 1). As can be seen from Table 1, performance outcome is systematically related to TRI in the anxious-defensive group only.

In addition, there was a positive correlation between CS and number of requests for relevant pieces of information (FRI) within both the anxious-defensive and anxious-sensitive groups, suggesting that the repeated preoccupation with task-relevant information was a valuable strategy for both groups. On the other hand, within the anxious-defensive group FRI was additionally related to TRI (see Table 1). The latter result may indicate that anxious-defensive subjects have limited resources to control their total amount of capacity available (see Kahneman, 1973, p. 15). This interpretation is supported by the self-report data. At the end of the experiment subjects were asked, "When your actual performance fell behind your normally available competence during the work, how often was this due to your inability to concentrate on task's demands?" (frequencies were rated on a 4-point scale; 1 = almost never, 4 = *almost always*). Anxious-defensive subjects scored significantly higher on this question than did anxious-sensitive and nonanxious subjects (anxious-defensive group—M = 3.18, SD = .88; anxious-sensitive group—M = 2.53, SD = 0.87; nonanxious group—M = 2.45, SD = 1.02), $F(2, 69)$ = 4.71, p < .01.

Information intake (time spent on problem identification), however, was found to correlate with correct solutions for both anxious-sensitive and anxious-defensive subjects. It appears, then, that what the anxious-sensitive and the anxious-defensive coping styles have in common is a short-term and intensified effort expenditure that results in enhanced performance. This regulatory process seems to be more effective for anxious-sensitive subjects than for anxious-defensive subjects, as their time-related efficiency is significantly higher (see Figure 4).

As regards the nonanxious subjects, there is only one substantial correlation (TRI × FRI) indicating that the more frequently relevant pieces of information were suggested, the longer the time spent on information processing. Finally, it seems worthwhile to mention that there were no significant differences in the means and standard deviations among the three groups with regard to the variables discussed earlier.

In sum, the data we have reported demonstrate that the anxious-sensitive and anxious-defensive coping styles, respectively, were associated with distinct characteristic patterns of behavior or action strategies (see also Moos & Billings, 1982).

Temporal Patterns of State Anxiety and the Macrostructure of Actions

The macrostructure of actions is here defined by (a) the different stages in the coping process relevant to task performance (e.g., anticipation, preparation, confrontation, and evaluation) and (b) the time structure or sequence of the tasks or action units that had to be performed. As mentioned earlier, the different stages in the coping process are reflected in the temporal patterns of state anxiety as presented in Figure 1. I now discuss the data with respect to the time structure or sequence of the eight blocks of tasks, where each block is considered to represent a separate action unit.

First, self-regulatory processes concerning the macrostructure of actions can be

Table 1 Correlations Between Number of Correct Solutions (CS), Time Spent on Problem Identification (TP), Time Spent on Relevant Pieces of Information (TRI), and Frequency of Relevant Pieces of Information (FRI) for Anxious-Defensive, Anxious-Sensitive and Nonanxious Subjects

	Anxious-defensive (n = 23)			Anxious-sensitive (n = 17)			Nonanxious (n = 32)		
	CS	TP	TRI	CS	TP	TRI	CS	TP	TRI
TP	− .45*	—		− .58*	—		.09	—	
TRI	.45*	− .11	—	− .07	.03	—	− .12	.07	—
FRI	.75**	− .27	.56**	.49*	− .42*	.38	.00	− .17	.35*

*p < .05.   **p < .01.

inferred from self-report data. Anxious-defensive subjects reported that they were not sufficiently able to concentrate on task-relevant information while performing the different blocks of tasks to a significantly higher degree than did the other two groups (anxious-defensive group—M = 20.2, SD = 3.57; anxious-sensitive group—M = 17.5, SD = 2.21; nonanxious group—M = 17.2, SD = 3.10; $F[2, 69]$ = 5.99, p <.001; where higher scores represent the inability to concentrate on task demands). A more detailed analysis of these data revealed that these differences between the groups were due mainly to the ratings at the end of the last three executed blocks of tasks, as during the execution of the first five blocks there were no significant differences among the three groups with regard to the ability to concentrate on task demands (see Figure 6).

Apparently, after they had worked about 2.5 hr on the tasks, failure feedback (subjects were informed about the performance level achieved at the end of each block), experienced fatigue, and corresponding increase of mental load led to concentration deficits in the anxious-defensive group (Figure 6).

In sum, these data provide further support for the contention that anxious-defensive subjects suffer from deficits in self-regulation (e.g., the internal regulation of activation, effort, or attention; see Bösel, 1986; Pribram & McGuinness, 1975; Sanders, 1983). Whereas these findings were primarily indicative for problem-focused coping strategies, emotion-focused coping strategies are considered in the next paragraph.

As can be seen from Figure 7, anxious-defensive subjects felt more emotionally disturbed than did anxious-sensitive subjects after finishing the last two blocks of tasks. Interestingly, however, these groups do not differ with respect to the sixth block. These findings may be explained as follows. Recall that the subjects had to interrupt their work after finishing the fifth block because of a forced rest pause that lasted about 15 min. For the anxious-defensive subjects, the rest pause may have been an opportunity to reestablish their defensive coping system (see Epstein, 1976), such that they again managed (see Houston, 1977, 1982) to divert attention from self-relevant threatening information during the sixth block. However, being confronted with "reality" for an even longer period of time, their coping system collapsed. For the anxious-sensitive group, in contrast, it seems reasonable to assume that their sensitive coping system (e.g., self-oriented cognitions or worries) had been activated during the rest pause. Because an anxious-sensitive coping style requires a comparatively large amount of time and the opportunity to actively master the tasks (see Krohne & Schaffner, 1980) in order to become effective in coping with self-related cognitions, anxious-sensitive subjects still responded with increased negative emotional states after they had finished the sixth block (i.e., the first block after the rest pause). Therefore, they experienced the same amount of negative feelings as the anxious-defensive subjects at this point of time. The same pattern of emotional states was found for the first three blocks of tasks (see Figure 7).

The motivational processes (see Heckhausen, 1982) during task execution are further elucidated by considering subjects' choice of tasks. As mentioned earlier, subjects had degrees of freedom with regard to the time and sequence in which they performed the different blocks of tasks. This is, they could, for example, start with easy blocks of tasks and finish with difficult ones, or vice versa.

Figure 8 shows the distribution of blocks of tasks in the course of the testing situation. As can be seen from Figure 8, there is a remarkable difference among

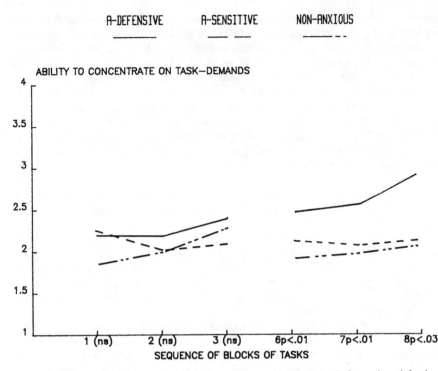

Figure 6 Subjective estimates of the ability to concentrate on task demands for anxious-defensive, anxious-sensitive, and nonanxious subjects.

the groups concerning their choice of tasks of different difficulty. Both the anxious-defensive and the nonanxious subjects preferred to begin with easy blocks of tasks. In contrast, the anxious-sensitive subjects preferred a more proportionate distribution. That is, the self-imposed task demands imposed in the first three blocks of tasks were significantly higher ($p < .01$) than those of the other two groups. Consequently, the task demands on the last three blocks of tasks were significantly lower ($p < .01$) for this group.

In sum, taking into account both the performance data and the self-report data concerning experienced states of stress, it can be stated that for both the anxious-sensitive and the nonanxious subjects, the preferred strategy on the level of the macrostructure of actions has proven to be efficient. In contrast, the results for anxious-defensive subjects (cf. Figure 8), indicating that they postponed difficult tasks, suggest that although these subjects initially profit from this strategy, when later confronted with more difficult tasks (see Figure 7, Blocks 3, 7, and 8), they fail to cope successfully.

CONCLUSIONS

This chapter emphasized the usefulness of an empirical exploration of different stages in an achievement-related stress situation. The study demonstrated that the relation between anxiety-related coping activities and goal-directed behavior varies depending on the following factors: (a) the temporal stage of the coping episode; (b) the choice, intensity, and flexibility of specific types of task-oriented and anxiety-related responses; (c) the nature of the stressor (e.g., task requirements and ego threat); (d) the performance criterion; (e) the person's capacity (e.g., ability and coping modes); and (f) the context of coping (e.g., situational demands and degrees of freedom with respect to individual planning and decision making).

Provided, as realized in this experiment, that the given task requirements remain constant, no time limit is imposed, and the task given offers degrees of freedom with respect to the duration and sequence of operations necessary for task solution, mental load as well as the corresponding stress responses are primarily determined by the relation between acquired coping styles and the efficiency of the activity structure (see Bachmann & Udris, 1982; Hacker, 1978, 1982; Schulz, 1982). Therefore, on the basis of the results reported in this chapter, it is suggested that anxiety-related coping strategies should be distinguished according to the functional role they play in different stages of the coping process. For instance, in the anticipation period (between task announcement and task application), avoidant thinking (Houston, 1977) or mental withdrawal (Carver & Scheier, 1982) may be effective in reducing anxiety and the costs of immediate effort expenditure (see Figure 2). During task execution (see Figures 6 and 7), in contrast, the same strategy may be inadequate (Epstein, 1976; Otto, 1981) in that it diverts attention away from task-relevant activities and thereby prevents the optimal allocation of

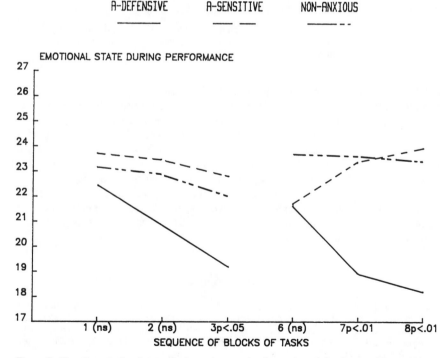

Figure 7 Negative emotional states during task execution for anxious-defensive, anxious-sensitive, and nonanxious subjects.

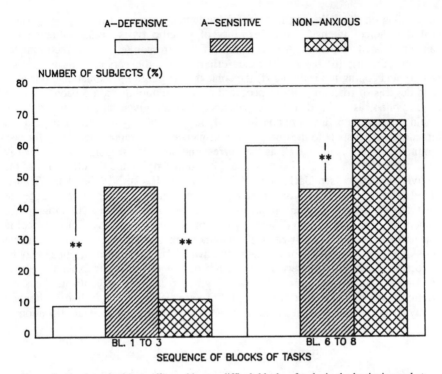

Figure 8 Number of subjects (%) working on difficult blocks of tasks in the beginning and at the end of the testing situation in the anxious-defensive, anxious-sensitive, and non-anxious groups.

available resources for meeting the task requirements (see Kahneman, 1973; Sanders, 1983; Schönpflug, 1983). Furthermore, the reported data suggest that a process-oriented approach or a transactional model (see Lazarus & Launier, 1978), that is, a model that takes into account personality variables (especially habitual coping modes) and situational variables, as well as task variables (e.g., cognitive requirements imposed on the subjects), offers a promising research strategy for the investigation of the mechanisms leading to states of stress and anxiety.

Although, obviously, further research is needed to elaborate on the conceptual outline proposed in this chapter, I believe that the empirical exploration of the coping process during different stages of a performance situation is essential to understanding the stress process.

REFERENCES

Asendorpf, J. B., Wallbott, H. G., & Scherer, K. R. (1983). Der verflixte Represser: Ein empirisch begründeter Vorschlag zu einer zweidimensionalen Operationalisierung von Repression-Sensitization. [The discrepant repressor: An empirically based proposal of a two dimensional approach to differentiate repressors and sensitizers]. *Zeitschrift für Differentielle und Diagnostische Psychologie, 4,* 113–128.
Bachmann, W., & Udris, I. (1982). *Mental load and stress in activity.* Amsterdam: North-Holland.

Bösel, R. (1986). Biopsychologie der emotionen [Biopsychology of emotions]. Berlin: Walter de Gruyter.

Carver, C. S., & Scheier, M. F. (1982). *Attention and self-regulation: A control-theory approach to human behavior.* New York: Springer-Verlag.

Epstein, S. (1976). Anxiety, arousal, and the self-concept. In C. D. Spielberger & I. G. Sarason (Eds.), *Stress and anxiety* (Vol. 3, pp. 185-224). New York: Wiley.

Eysenck, M. W. (1982). *Attention and arousal.* New York: Springer-Verlag.

Hacker, W. (1978). *Allgemeine Ingenieur-und Arbeitspsychologie.* [Engineering and work psychology]. Berlin, German Democratic Republic: Deutscher Verlag der Wissenschaften.

Hacker, W. (1982). Objective and subjective organization of work activities. In M. von Cranach & R. Hare (Eds.), *The analysis of action.* (pp. 73-91). Cambridge, England: Cambridge University Press.

Heckhausen, H. (1982). Task irrelevant cognitions during an exam: Incidence and effects. In H. W. Krohne & L. Laux (Eds.), *Achievement, stress, and anxiety* (pp. 247-274). Washington, DC: Hemisphere.

Houston, B. K. (1977). Dispositional anxiety and the effectiveness of cognitive coping strategies in stressful laboratory and classroom situations. In C. D. Spielberger & I. G. Sarason (Eds.), *Stress and anxiety* (Vol. 4, pp. 205-226). Washington, DC: Hemisphere.

Houston, B. K. (1982). Trait anxiety and cognitive coping behavior. In H. W. Krohne & L. Laux (Eds.), *Achievement, stress, and anxiety* (pp. 195-206). Washington, DC: Hemisphere.

Janis, I. L. (1982). Decisionmaking under stress. In L. Goldberger & S. Breznitz (Eds.), *Handbook of stress* (pp. 69-87). New York: Free Press.

Kahneman, D. (1973). *Attention and effort.* Englewood Cliffs, NJ: Prentice-Hall.

Krohne, H. W., & Rogner, P. (1982). Repression-sensitization as a central construct in coping research. In H. W. Krohne & L. Laux (Eds.), *Achievement, stress, and anxiety* (pp. 167-193). Washington, DC: Hemisphere.

Krohne, H. W., & Schaffner, P. (1980, June). *Anxiety, coping strategies, and test performance.* Invited paper presented at the Fourth International Symposium on Educational Testing, Antwerp, Belgium.

Laux, L., Glanzmann, P., Schaffner, P., & Spielberger, C. D. (1981). *Das State-Trait-Inventar* [The State-Trait Inventory]. Weinheim: Beltz.

Laux, L., & Vossel, G. (1982). Paradigms in stress research: Laboratory versus field and traits versus processes. In L. Goldberger & S. Breznitz (Eds.), *Handbook of stress: Theoretical and clinical aspects.* (pp. 203-211). New York: Free Press.

Lazarus, R. S., & Launier, R. (1978). Stress-related transactions between person and environment. In L. A. Pervin & M. Lewis (Eds.), *Perspectives in interactional psychology.* New York: Plenum Press.

Moos, R. H., & Billings, A. G. (1982). Conceptualizing and measuring coping resources and process. In L. Goldberger & S. Breznitz (Eds.), *Handbook of stress: Theoretical and clinical aspects.* (pp. 213-230). New York: Free Press.

Otto, J. (1981). *Regulationsmuster in Warte- und Vollzugssituationen.* [Regulatory activity during waiting and performance]. Munich, Federal Republic of Germany: Mineerva.

Pribram, K. H., & McGuinness, D. (1975). Arousal, activation, and effort in the control of attention. *Psychological Review, 82,* 116-149.

Sanders, A. F. (1983). Towards a model of stress and human performance. *Acta Psychologica, 53,* 61-97.

Schönpflug, W. (1983). Coping efficiency and situational demands. In G. R. Hockey (Ed.), *Stress and fatigue in human performance.* (pp. 299-330). London: Wiley.

Schönpflug, W., & Battmann, W. (1982). *Psychologische Effekte bei Langzeiteinwirkung von Verkehrslärm* [Psychological effects of long term traffic noise]. (Forschungsbericht Nr. 82-10501 304). Berlin, Federal Republic of Germany: Umweltbundesamt.

Schönpflug, W., & Schulz, P. (1979). *Lärmwirkungen bei Tätigkeiten mit komplexer Informationsverarbeitung* [The impact of noise on complex information processing]. (Forschungsbericht Nr. 79-10501 201). Berlin, Federal Republic of Germany: Umweltbundesamt.

Schönpflug, W., & Wieland, R. (1982). *Schwankende Schallpegel Leistungshandeln und der Wechsel von Arbeit und Erholung* [Oscillating sound levels, performance and the change between work and recreation] (Forschungsbericht Nr. 82-10501 204). Berlin, Federal Republic of Germany: Umweltbundesamt.

Schulz, P. (1982). Mental and emotional load in goal-directed behavior. In W. Bachmann & I. Udris (Eds.), *Mental load and stress in activity.* (pp. 69-78). Amsterdam: North-Holland.

Schulz, P., & Battmann, W. (1980). Die Auswirkungen von Verkehrslärm auf verschiedene Tätigkeiten. *Zeitschrift für experimentelle und angewandte Psychologie* [The impact of traffic noise on different activities], 27, 592–606.

Schulz, P., & Schönpflug, W. (1982). Regulatory activity during states of stress. In H. W. Krohne & L. Laux (Eds.), *Achievement, stress, and anxiety* (pp. 51–73). Washington, DC: Hemisphere.

Spielberger, C. D. (1972). Anxiety as an emotional state. In C. D. Spielberger (Ed.), *Anxiety: Current trends in theory and research* (Vol. 1, pp. 23–44). New York: Academic Press.

Spielberger, C. D. (1975). Anxiety: State-trait-process. In C. D. Spielberger & I. G. Sarason (Eds.), *Stress and anxiety* (Vol. 1, pp. 115–143). New York: Wiley.

Weinberger, D. A., Schwartz, G. E., & Davidson, R. J. (1979). Low-anxious, high-anxious, and repressive coping styles: Psychometric patterns and behavioral and physiological responses to stress. *Journal of Abnormal Psychology, 88,* 369–380.

Weiner, H. (1982). An attribution theory of motivation and emotion. In H. W. Krohne & L. Laux (Eds.), *Achievement, stress, and anxiety* (pp. 223–245). Washington, DC: Hemisphere.

Wieland, R. (1981). Schwankende Schallpegel, Leistungshandeln und der Wechsel von Arbeit und Erholung. [Oscillating sound levels, performance and the work recreation cycle] *Zeitschrift für Lärmbekämpfung, 25,* 117–122.

Wieland, R. (1984). Temporal patterns of anxiety: Towards a process analysis of anxiety and performance. In R. Schwarzer (Ed.), *The self in anxiety, stress, and depression.* (pp. 133–150). Amsterdam: North-Holland.

8

Depression and Test Anxiety in Comprehension and Memory: Independent Effects?

John J. Hedl, Jr.
*University of Texas
Southwestern Medical Center at Dallas, USA*

James C. Bartlett
University of Texas at Dallas, USA

This chapter examines depression, state test anxiety (worry), and comprehension effects in sentence memory as a function of imagery and semantic encoding strategies. Across two experiments with college students, negative depression effects were consistently found with a semantic encoding strategy, but not with an imagery strategy. If anything, the state worry effects were stronger with an imagery strategy. Importantly, the relation between depression and anxiety varied by encoding condition, supporting speculation that encoding tasks can alter the relation of depression and cognitive worry. Imagery encoding conditions attenuated the depression effects; semantic encoding conditions did not. The hypothesis that effects on memory are mediated by comprehension failures was supported more clearly for state test anxiety than for depression. The pattern of evidence favors a cognitive interference model of depression, with cognitive worry as an important component.

In the general experimental literature, the effects of emotional states (e.g., depression, elation, sadness, etc.) on memory are currently receiving a great deal of attention (e.g., Bower, 1981; Ellis, Thomas, & Rodriquez, 1984; Leight & Ellis, 1981). In the test anxiety literature, an impressive body of evidence suggests that detrimental effects of test anxiety on learning, memory, and performance exist, can be demonstrated in educational and laboratory settings across elementary school through college, and are particularly robust under conditions of evaluative stress and failure (Krohne & Laux, 1982; Sarason, 1980; Schwarzer, van der Ploeg, & Spielberger, 1982, 1987; van der Ploeg, Schwarzer, & Spielberger, 1983–1985). Interest in depression topics such as learned helplessness is being

We thank Patsy Moore and Karen Hatchett for typing and editing and other clerical work associated with these studies. Frank Burns was very helpful in conducting the student sessions and with data reduction activities. Kent Dana was very helpful with advice on various statistical analyses and computer procedures. Portions of the project were supported with institutional research grant funds to John J. Hedl.

seen among test anxiety researchers as well (Schwarzer, Jerusalem, & Schwarzer, 1983; Schwarzer, Jerusalem, & Stiksrud, 1984). There is now considerable evidence that variables related to anxiety, depression, and other emotional states can influence the efficiency of mnemonic functioning (see Eysenck, 1982; Hasher & Zacks, 1979) as well as the qualitative aspects of such functioning (see Bower, 1981). However, little is still known concerning the principles that govern the appearance of such effects, the mechanisms through which they occur (e.g., elaboration, distinctiveness, effort, self-cognitions, motivation, etc.), or how different emotional states compare (such as anxiety and depression).

The present research was primarily concerned with the effects of depression on comprehension and memory for meaningful sentence materials. To study this area, we adopted a research paradigm developed by Till (1977; Till, Cormak, & Prince, 1977) and others (e.g., Auble & Franks, 1978; Johnson, Bransford, & Soloman, 1973) that has recently been applied to the problem of memory aging (Till, 1985; Till & Walsh, 1980). This paradigm involves testing memory for sentences for which comprehension is effortful in that it depends on inferring information not explicitly stated. For example, "The general raised his glass in the air" is an example of a sentence that can be interpreted as a "toast," but only by going beyond the information given in the sentence. Memory for such sentences can be tested in response to inferential cues (e.g., *toast* in the preceding example). Recall of sentences in response to such cues has been shown to be sensitive to manipulations of semantic processing at input (Till et al., 1977). Thus, recall of sentences to inferential cues apparently is reflective of comprehension of these sentences at input.

Some prior experiments we have done in the test anxiety area (Hedl & Bartlett, 1981, 1982, 1985, 1989) have corroborated the importance of comprehension processes for inference-cued recall and recognition of sentences, and have suggested the hypothesis that comprehension can mediate test anxiety–sentence memory relations. In these experiments, we asked our subjects to respond to each of the sentences in an input list by writing a word or phrase conveying their understanding of it (cf. Till & Walsh, 1980). We scored each response as indicating an appropriate inference or not. Sentence comprehension as scored in this manner was strongly associated with subsequent recall of the sentences. Furthermore, measures of state test anxiety were reliably correlated with sentence comprehension and sentence recall.

Our major goal in the present experiments was to extend our prior test anxiety research to the depression area and direct it toward three issues. First, can depression–memory relations be explained partly by depression–comprehension relations similar to those for test anxiety–memory? Or do the links between depression and other memory processes appear to be more critical? Second, does the encoding strategy used mediate depression–memory relations? Third, do state test anxiety and memory relations replicate our previous experiments? The uniformity of depression and anxiety effects was an additional question of interest.

Our primary encoding comparison was between imagery and semantic instructions. Imagery was of concern for several reasons. First, our previous research with this paradigm suggested that imagery is a useful strategy (Hedl & Bartlett, 1982). Following a sentence-memory experiment in which they were not given a specific encoding strategy to use, students were asked to describe the strategy(ies) they used to learn the sentences during the input phase of the experiment. In a series of post hoc analyses, students who reported the use of an imagery strategy showed superior free recall and cued recall of the sentences as compared with verbal elaboration, physical strategy, rote, or no strategy (see Weinstein, Underwood, Wicker, & Cubberly, 1979, for a description of this classification scheme in the learning strategy area). However, the sample size did not permit a useful analysis for possible relations with levels of state test anxiety and strategy use.

Second, other researchers have demonstrated the positive effects of imagery across laboratory and educational settings (cf. Levin, 1981; Paivio & Descrochers, 1981; Peters, Levin, McGivern, & Pressley, 1985). In the trait-anxiety area, Edmunsen and Nelson (1976) have reported that an imagery strategy was beneficial for high-anxious students in a paired-associate experiment. Imagery can be found in a number of learning strategy programs (O'Neil, 1978; O'Neil & Spielberger, 1979). A recent publication summarizes much of the research on imagery and education (Sheikh & Sheikh, 1985). In general, for adults and for children in second grade and beyond, verbal instructions to form mental images of paired associates, sentences, or even longer prose passages have improved both recognition and recall. The majority of these studies compared imagery with verbal rehearsal or other shallow encoding processes. The effectiveness of imagery as compared with other elaborative encoding processes remains an open question, particularly in the sentence-memory area (Pressley, Symons, McDaniel, Snyder, & Turnure, 1988).

Depression was of interest because of the recent growth in research on the effects of mood states on learning and memory. It has been proposed that the debilitating effects of a depressed mood state are greater when the processing involved in a task is more complex and demanding (Ellis et al., 1984; Ellis, Thomas, McFarland, & Lane, 1985). This predicted interaction between depressed mood states and encoding difficulty has some empirical support (e.g., Ellis et al., 1984, Experiments 1 and 3; Hasher & Zacks, 1979). However, an open question is whether complex encoding processes that are beneficial to memory decrease depression effects on memory. Imagery might be such a complex, efficacious process.

An equally important issue is whether anxiety and depression affect memory in similar ways. If depression and test anxiety yield similar effects on memory, the suggestion would be that they have an impact on common memorial processes such as comprehension. If, however, the effects of these two variables differ qualitatively—possibly as a function of encoding strategy—then this would be evidence that these emotional states affect different cognitive processes (e.g, attention, cognitive effort, etc.). Although the two encoding strategies of interest here (imagery or semantic) may not differ in terms of recall for normal populations, clinical research suggests that imagery might lessen the short-term effects of depression (Schultz, 1978). The exact mechanism(s) underlying the imagery effect in these situations is not at all well understood (e.g., change in encoding strategy, decrease in negative self-talk, etc.).

Although our primary concerns were with comprehension and cued recall, we administered a test of sentence free recall. The purpose of including free recall was based on the finding of Till and Walsh (1980) that, under some encoding conditions, differences between young and elderly adults are not found in cued recall of sentences, although they are present in free recall of sentences. Although age-related differences and depression- or anxiety-related differences may or may not have similar causes, the Till and Walsh findings raise the possibility of no effects of a variable in cued recall but significant effects in free recall, a possibility that seemed worthwhile to assess.

EXPERIMENT 1

Method

Subjects

Forty-one female volunteers from introductory psychology classes were randomly assigned to imagery ($n = 21$) or semantic ($n = 20$) encoding strategies. They received course credit for their participation.

Personality Measures

The Beck Depression Inventory (BDI; Beck, Ward, Mendelson, Mock, & Erbaugh, 1961) was used to measure level of depression. The BDI is a clinically derived self-report inventory of depression for use with psychiatric populations. It was constructed to assess the current depth of depression, whether depression is viewed as the primary diagnosis or not. It consists of 21 items covering affective, cognitive, motivational, and physiological areas of depressive symptomatology. Bumberry, Oliver, and McClure (1978) have reported concurrent validity with psychiatric ratings of depression with a college student population. Furthermore, the BDI is a widely used instrument in the study of psychological deficit (e.g., Miller, 1975) and is in current use in studying the effects of emotion and cognition with college students (cf. Hasher, Rose, Zacks, Sanft, & Doren, 1985).

The revised version of the Worry-Emotionality Questionnaire (WEQ; Morris, Davis, and Hutchings, 1981) was used to measure levels of state test anxiety. The WEQ yields subscale scores for worry and emotionality. Worry refers to the intensity of the students' cognitive concern about their performance and emotionality refers to perceptions of physiological arousal.

Experimental Materials

A set of 24 sentences, including 4 filler sentences to control for primacy and recency effects, was taken from previous research (Hedl & Bartlett, 1981, 1982). These sentences, modeled after Till et al. (1977) and Auble, Franks, and Soraci (1979), were of the form

> The house turned to water because the fire got too hot.
> The general raised his glass in the air.

These sentences were developed such that certain inferences or elaborations would be probable for the student engaged in an elaborate semantic processing strategy (Craik & Tulving, 1975). Recall was tested with inference cues: *igloo* was the inference cue for the first example: *toast* was the inference cue for the second.

Procedure

The experiment was conducted with small groups (about 8–10 people per session). After being given a brief, general orientation the students completed the BDI. All students were told that the experiment was concerned with how college students learn and remember sentences. They were given either imagery or semantic encoding instructions. For imagery, they were told that mental imagery was an excellent strategy for learning sentences. As they listened to each sentence, they were to try to form a picture of the sentence situation or event. For the semantic instructions, students were told to think about the event being described in each sentence and the things that might be involved in this event. Two example sentences were provided in each condition. Both sets of students were to write down a word or phrase as a response to their interpretation of the sentence. The sentences were read aloud by the experimenter at the rate of one new sentence every 10 s. Each sentence was presented and immediately repeated to minimize errors of speech perception.

After presentation of the 24 sentences, students performed a writing-speed task. They were told to write down as many numbers as they could beginning with 100 and proceeding backwards. Students were then given approximately 5–6 min for free recall.[1]

The final test was a cued-recall test consisting of inference cues. Students were told of this cue type and shown two sentence examples along with cues. The experimenter then read each inference cue aloud and allowed 30 s for the subjects' written response.

Using procedures similar to our previous experiments, students completed the (WEQ) with retrospective state instructions. Students were then asked to rate the amount of time they spent "concentrating" on the sentences during the initial presentation, using an 11-point scale (0%–100%). All students were then debriefed and given the opportunity to ask any questions.

Comprehension and Sentence Scoring

In terms of scoring, comprehension scores at encoding were derived from students' written responses to sentences from the input list. These comprehension responses were scored as correct if the students listed the main inference (*toast*) or one that represented some understanding of the sentence (e.g., *party, honor*). Two raters showed a reliability of .91 for the comprehension scores for a subset of the data. Free- and cued-recall sentence responses were scored in terms of the lenient criteria established by Till et al. (1977).[2] That is, sentences were scored as correct if they were recalled verbatim, contained synonymous substitutions or omissions of partially redundant information, or specified the agent, verb, and some additional information. For a subset of the sentence-recall data, reliability of two raters was .96 in Experiment 1; it was equally as high in the second experiment.

Results

Given the continuous nature of the depression and state test anxiety indices, and the relatively small sample size within encoding conditions, the primary analytic approach was to examine the magnitude and direction of the correlations among depression, state test anxiety, comprehension, and memory performance separately as a function of the two encoding task conditions. Multiple regression analyses

---

[1]Our previous studies have shown this time limit to be quite adequate for free recall in this task with college students.

[2]Analyses were also performed by using a strict scoring criterion for sentence recall, and the same pattern of results was found in both free recall and cued recall in both experiments. As expected, strict scoring led to lower scores for all students. The correlations between the two derived scores were high (.90 and beyond), and analyses with the personality measures yielded similar outcomes across studies.

were then computed to corroborate the interpretation of the varying bivariate relations.

Comparison of Imagery and Semantic Strategies

A preliminary set of analyses examined the memory performance and personality measures as a function of encoding task. As presented in Table 1, the two groups were markedly similar on all but one variable ($ts < 1$). Students in the imagery condition reported significantly higher levels of concentration at encoding (67%) than those who received semantic instructions (54%), a marginally significant effect ($p < .10$). The lack of significant differences in recall between imagery and semantic encoding strategies is consistent with prior research on adults (Pressley et al., 1988).

Depression and Comprehension

A first point to be made concerns the relation of sentence comprehension to level of depression. Depression scores were not significantly correlated with comprehension scores in either encoding condition (second column of Table 2), although the correlation was positive in the imagery condition and negative in the semantic one. Comprehension was, however, strongly related to subsequent recall performance. For all subjects, the correlation between scored comprehension at input and free recall was .54 ($p < .01$); it was .74 ($p < .01$) for cued recall. This pattern was maintained when the correlations were examined within both encoding groups (see Table 2, Rows 4 and 8).

Depression and Memory

In terms of BDI depression scores, an interesting pattern of correlations emerged between the two encoding conditions (see Table 2, Rows 1 and 4). In the

Table 1 Comparison of Imagery and Semantic Encoding Task Conditions: Experiment 1

Measures	Encoding strategy				
	Imagery ($n = 21$)		Semantic ($n = 20$)		
	M	SD	M	SD	t
Memory performance					
Comprehension	9.48	3.93	9.50	3.90	0.01
Free recall	6.29	2.90	5.90	2.43	0.46
Cued recall	10.29	4.34	10.10	4.34	0.14
Personality measures					
Depression (Beck Depression Inventory)	7.00	7.90	9.90	6.67	−1.27
Worry (Worry-Emotionality Questionnaire)	9.38	2.97	10.20	4.34	−0.71
Emotionality (Worry-Emotionality Questionnaire)	6.57	1.94	5.95	1.15	1.24
Other measures					
Concentration	67%	.23	54%	.25	1.73*

*$p < .10$, two-tailed.

Table 2 Correlations of Depression, State Test Anxiety, and Memory within Encoding Task Condition

Condition	Comprehension	Free recall	Cued recall
Imagery encoding condition (n = 21)			
Depression	.22	.40***	.46*
	(.11)	(.26)	(.35)
WEQ Worry	−.38	−.64**	−.57**
	(−.33)	(−.59)**	(−.50)*
WEQ Emotionality	.15	−.41***	−.28
	(.28)	(−.33)	(−.16)
Comprehension	—	.59**	.71**
Semantic encoding condition (n = 20)			
Depression	−.12	−.62**	−.48*
	(.10)	(−.18)	(−.00)
WEQ Worry	−.24	−.70**	−.61**
	(−.23)	(−.44)*	(−.43)***
WEQ Emotionality	−.33	−.29	−.25
	(−.28)	(−.16)	(−.12)
Comprehension	—	.49*	.77**

Note. WEQ = Worry-Emotionality Questionnaire. Partial correlations are given in parentheses. For depression–memory correlations, WEQ worry was partialed; for WEQ worry–memory correlations, depression was removed; for WEQ emotionality–memory correlations, WEQ worry was removed.
*p < .05. **p < .01. ***p < .10.

imagery condition, we note a significant positive correlation between BDI scores and memory. The overall correlation was marginally significant for free recall (p < .07) and significant for inference-cued recall (r = .46, p < .05). In contrast, level of depression was negatively related to both free recall (r = −.62, p < .01) and inference-cued recall (r = −.48, p < .05) within the semantic encoding condition.

The varying pattern of depression–memory correlations by encoding condition was buttressed by a series of multiple regression analyses that examined comprehension, free recall, and inference-cued recall as a function of level of depression, encoding strategy (coded as 0 for imagery, 1 for semantic), and their interaction. For comprehension, no significant effects were found. For free recall, however, the overall model was significant, $F(7, 33) = 7.02, p < .0001$, and significant effects were found for depression ($t = 2.2, p < .04$), strategy ($t = 2.4, p < .02$), and the Depression × Strategy interaction ($t = −3.55, p < .001$). The same pattern of significant effects was found for inference-cued recall.

An additional set of regression analyses included scored comprehension as a factor for both free recall and cued recall. The important point to note here is that the depression effects found previously remained reliable with comprehension in the model. Additionally, comprehension was reliably associated with free and cued recall, and entered into interactions with depression and strategy. (In fact, the only nonsignificant effect in both analyses was the Strategy × Encoding interaction in cued recall.)

State Test Anxiety and Memory Performance

The correlations between WEQ state test anxiety scores and memory performance are presented in Table 2 separately for the two encoding conditions.[3] Considering free recall and inference-cued recall, a consistent pattern of test anxiety and performance correlations was found. State test worry was reliably (and negatively) related to free recall and cued recall in both the imagery and semantic encoding conditions (all $ps < .01$). The magnitude of these free and cued recall correlations with worry was not found to differ significantly in either encoding condition. None of the four state worry or emotionality correlations with comprehension were significant (see second column of Table 2).

Similar to the depression analyses, multiple regression analyses were conducted to examine worry effects between the two encoding conditions. Congruent with the depression findings, comprehension was unrelated to worry, encoding strategy, or their interaction. For free and cued recall, however, the pattern was different from that of depression. Here were found only main effects for worry in both analyses; specifically, there were no worry–strategy interactions.

Another discrepancy between the depression and test anxiety findings emerged in the regression analyses. When comprehension was included in the model, the worry effect did not reach conventional significance levels in cued recall, although it remained reliable in free recall. Thus, the cued-recall evidence suggests that worry effects, unlike depression effects, were mediated by comprehension to some degree.

The independence of the anxiety and depression effects can be seen clearly by examining the intercorrelations of the depression and anxiety measures in each condition. In the imagery condition, depression scores were not correlated significantly with either WEQ worry ($r = -.33$) or WEQ emotionality ($r = -.18$). For the semantic condition, however, depression scores were reliably related to worry ($r = .76, p < .01$) but not to emotionality ($r = .21$).

Given this pattern of depression–anxiety correlations, we examined partial correlations within the two encoding conditions. These are reported in Table 2 in parentheses. In the imagery condition, the depression and memory performance correlations were reduced, but remained positive when worry was partialed out. The worry–memory correlations remained reliable when depression was partialed out. In the semantic condition, however, depression–memory correlations were eliminated when worry was taken into account. The worry–memory correlations remained robust when depression scores were taken into consideration, however.

Summary

The primary question addressed in Experiment 1 was whether depression effects could be demonstrated in long-term sentence memory and whether the relation would vary as a function of the encoding strategy used. An additional question

---

[3]In general, level of test anxiety as measured by the Test Anxiety Inventory (TAI; Spielberger, 1980) was unrelated to memory performance in these studies and generally in the previous studies that used similar sentence materials and procedures (see Hedl & Bartlett, 1981, 1982, 1985, 1989). Only the state measures of test anxiety (primarily worry) were found to be consistently associated with memory performance.

was concerned with how depression and anxiety compare in their effects on memory.

Regarding the first question, depression was positively related to free and cued recall in the imagery strategy condition, but negatively related in the semantic strategy condition. The negative depression effect in the semantic encoding condition is consistent with prior literature using both normal and clinical samples (Miller, 1975; however, see Hasher et al., 1985, for nonsignificant depression effects). However, the positive relation between depression and memory performance in the imagery condition is a more unusual finding. It is not typical of previous findings in the depression area; it does not appear to be explainable from either a resource allocation model or a schema theory of mood effects; and it is not expected from cognitive theories of depression relating depressed mood states to cognitive functioning (e.g., Beck, 1967).

What then can account for the finding of a positive relation between depression and inference-cue test performance in the imagery condition? First, from a pessimistic perspective, it is possible that the effect is due to sampling error and will not replicate. The sample size from the experiment was modest. The second point is suggested by the varying correlations between depression and anxiety by encoding condition. In the imagery condition, the correlation between depression and anxiety was negative; in the semantic condition, it was positive. This pattern suggests that perhaps the imagery task served to reduce cognitive worry. That is, depression may lead to reduced task performance, but only when depression is linked to worry. It is consistent with this speculation that the partial correlations showed that depression–memory relations were reduced (imagery condition) or eliminated (semantic condition) when worry was removed.

The second study we report tests the replicability of these patterns, using a similar, yet altered, sentence-memory experimental paradigm. Furthermore, this refined paradigm enabled us to explore the possibility that post-comprehension processes found to be an important predictor of memory processes are a factor in depression or test anxiety as well.

EXPERIMENT 2

This study was initially directed toward examining whether effort toward comprehension is a factor in effects of depression on memory. In the domain of sentence memory, Auble and Franks (1978) and Auble et al. (1979) developed a paradigm that enables a comparison of both comprehension and effort toward comprehension as factors in sentence recall. These authors have shown that the free recall of difficult-to-interpret sentences (such as those used in Experiment 1) is improved under conditions in which subjects actively attempt to interpret the sentences, as opposed to conditions in which "cues" for the correct interpretation are embedded within the sentence itself.

Consider, for example, the following sentence used in Experiment 1: "The haystack was important because the cloth ripped." This difficult-to-interpret sentence could be presented as is (no cue) or with a cue embedded within it to make it comprehensible (and low effort), as in "The haystack was important because the cloth of the parachute ripped." This sentence could also be presented in a high-effort mode with the cue *parachute* being presented 5 s after the initial presentation of the core sentence. Data from a number of experiments by Auble and her colleagues (Auble & Franks, 1978; Auble et al., 1979) indicated that free-recall performance was higher in the delayed-cue condition (high effort) than in the embedded-cue condition (low effort), suggesting that effort toward comprehension has a positive effect on memory performance independent of comprehension. Data from the no-cue condition showed that cognitive effort was not beneficial unless comprehension of the sentence was ultimately achieved.

In Experiment 2, we questioned whether effort toward comprehension alters the effects of depression or test anxiety on memory. Of greater importance here, we included a between-subjects comparison of encoding strategy: a semantic encoding strategy versus an imagery strategy. Thus, a partial replication of the imagery findings from Experiment 1 is possible. As before, we also included measures of state test anxiety to continue our comparisons of the differential effects of these two emotional states on sentence-memory processes.

Method

Subjects

Subjects were 84 female volunteers from introductory psychology classes at a metropolitan university who received course credit for their participation. They were randomly assigned to the six experimental conditions: Strategy (semantic vs. semantic plus imagery) × Input List (three counterbalanced versions). The experiment was run in groups of 6–8 students.

Materials and Procedures

The experiment was conducted by using a set of 27 sentences, 18 of which were used in previous experiments (Hedl & Bartlett, 1981, 1982) and 9 that were selected from Auble et al. (1979). The first and last two sentences in the list were filler items designed to reduce primacy and recency effects in the target list of 24 sentences. They were not used in the statistical analyses. One third of the sentences were not presented with a cue, and one third had the cue embedded in the sentence. The remaining one third were presented with a cue after a 5-s delay. The three types of sentences were randomly intermixed during the initial presentation. Three different input lists were formed and counterbalanced such that each sentence appeared with no cue, with an embedded cue, or with a postcue in equal numbers in both the imagery and semantic orienting task conditions.

Students were told that the sentences would vary in comprehensiveness and that some of the sentences would be followed by a word that might help the subjects to understand the sentence. Students in the imagery condition were given additional instructions to develop a picture of the sentence situation or event that incorporated all of the major objects included in the sentence. Two example sentences were then presented in both encoding task conditions.

After presentation of each sentence–cue combination and the 5-s delay, the experimenter said "Mark," and the students rated whether they understood the sentence, did not understand the sentence, or were unsure whether they understood the sentence. They were given 2 s to rate each sentence before the next sentence was presented.

Consistent with Experiment 1, students were given a writing-speed task followed by 5 min for free recall. An inference-cue test was then administered, the design of which followed similar counterbalancing considerations used in Experiment 1. Following cued recall, students completed the WEQ with instructions to indicate their feelings during the experiment. All students were then debriefed and given the opportunity to ask questions about the experiment.

Results

Because the second study had considerably more subjects (84 vs. 41), a more refined analytic approach was possible. Here three levels of depression (low, mild, and moderate) were examined, using cut-off scores derived from the clinical depression literature, not merely a tripartite split of the observed depression scores within an experiment (see Beck et al., 1961). Prior research has shown the importance of such an approach (see review by Miller, 1975). The second between-subjects factor was encoding strategy (imagery or semantic). Analyses focused on comprehension, free recall, and cued recall and were followed by post hoc examination of the depression and anxiety effects within encoding task condition.

Comparison of Imagery and Semantic Conditions

Preliminary analyses examined the memory performance and personality measures as a function of encoding condition. The means and standard deviations of these measures are reported in Table 3. Generally, as with Experiment 1, the two conditions were relatively equivalent on the majority of measures. We did note that the imagery condition led to higher self-ratings of comprehension and that the

Table 3 Comparison of Imagery and Semantic Encoding Task Conditions: Experiment 2

| | Encoding strategy | | | | |
| | Imagery (n = 42) | | Semantic (n = 42) | | |
Measures	M	SD	M	SD	t
Memory performance					
Comprehension (self-ratings)	19.9	2.6	18.57	2.61	2.34*
Free recall[a]	6.45	2.48	6.17	2.74	0.49
Cued recall	17.26	3.48	16.74	4.28	0.61
Personality measures					
Depression (Beck Depression Inventory)	9.86	7.24	8.52	6.33	0.90
Worry (Worry-Emotionality Questionnaire)	9.38	3.17	8.83	3.18	0.79
Emotionality (Worry-Emotionality Questionnaire)	6.71	2.21	6.75	2.67	−0.07
Other measures					
Concentration	58%	0.25	48%	0.24	1.87**

[a]For free- and cued-recall comparisons of the no cue, postcue, and embedded cue, mean differences between encoding conditions were uniformly not significant.
*p < .05. **p < .10.

mean "concentration" ratings for the imagery condition were again higher, although only marginally significant in this experiment.

The means and standard deviations of the comprehension, free-recall, and cued-recall measures are given in Table 4 as a function of encoding condition, level of depression, and state test worry.

Depression and Comprehension

The analyses of the self-ratings of comprehension (as compared with an actual scored measure of comprehension in Experiment 1) did not yield any main effects for level of depression or encoding strategy, and did not yield any interaction. There was a main effect for type of cue (no cue, postcue, or embedded cue); this indicated that the two cue conditions had similar levels of self-rated comprehension (92% vs. 91%), which were both higher than the ratings for the no-cue sentences (58%). These subjective, introspective self-ratings of comprehension were unrelated to memory performance, in marked contrast to those comprehension–memory relations noted in Experiment 1 for an actual scored measure of comprehension.

Depression and Memory

The free-recall analysis of variance (ANOVA; repeated measures, unweighted means solution) produced a significant effect for type of sentence cue (no cue, postcue, embedded cue), $F(2, 156) = 44.74, p < .0001$. Of greater interest here, we found a marginally significant interaction ($p < .06$) between level of depression and encoding strategy. To analyze this interaction further, two additional one-way ANOVAs were performed to examine depression effects in the imagery and semantic encoding strategy conditions separately. In the imagery condition, the ANOVA was not significant and indicated the lack of depression effects (see Table 4). In contrast, the effect of depression in the semantic encoding strategy was marginally significant, $F(2, 39) = 2.61, p < .08$, and suggested that the poorest performance was noted by the group with the moderate level of depression (18%), with the highest level of free-recall performance seen in the mildly depressed group (31%). The low depressed group showed performance levels in between those of the moderate and low depressed groups (26%).

The inference-cued-recall data were also analyzed as a function of depression, strategy, and type of cue. In this $3 \times 2 \times 3$ ANOVA we noted a significant depression main effect, $F(2, 28) = 5.02, p < .01$; a main effect for type of cue, $F(2, 156) = 128.49, p < .001$; and a marginal ($p < .08$) interaction between type of encoding cue and encoding strategy. In general, the imagery condition, compared with the semantic one, led to higher performance for the postcue sentences (87% vs. 77%), but did not appear to make any difference for the no-cue or embedded-cue conditions, regardless of encoding-cue condition (45% vs. 46%).

Although we found no Depression × Strategy interaction, a one-way ANOVA for the imagery condition showed no significant depression effect, $F(2, 39) = 1.01$, whereas a one-way ANOVA of the semantic condition cued-recall data yielded a significant effect of depression, $F(2, 39) = 4.19, p < .03$. In this latter case, the moderately depressed subjects showed the lowest performance (53%) and the low and mild groups were generally equivalent (71% vs. 77%).

Table 4   Means and Standard Deviations of Memory Performance by Level of Depression, Test
Anxiety, and Encoding Condition: Experiment 2

Encoding Condition	Comprehension[a]		Free recall		Cued recall	
	M	SD	M	SD	M	SD
Imagery encoding condition (n = 42)						
Depression						
Low (n = 23)	20.13	2.74	6.91	2.79	17.52	3.33
Mild (n = 11)	20.45	2.07	5.55	1.86	17.91	3.24
Moderate (n = 8)	19.00	2.73	6.37	2.13	15.75	4.17
State test worry						
Low (n = 13)	21.31	1.84	8.00	2.16	19.85	2.04
Mild (n = 16)	19.68	2.98	6.38	2.65	17.18	3.01
High (n = 13)	19.07	2.25	5.00	1.63	14.85	3.48
Semantic encoding condition (n = 42)						
Depression						
Low (n = 26)	18.62	3.11	6.19	2.68	16.96	3.79
Mid (n = 10)	18.40	1.35	7.50	2.12	18.50	2.37
Moderate (n = 6)	18.67	1.97	4.33	3.50	12.66	4.36
State test worry						
Low (n = 11)	19.67	1.91	7.00	2.93	18.80	3.45
Mid (n = 16)	18.56	2.37	5.88	2.92	15.75	3.66
High (n = 15)	17.09	3.18	5.72	2.41	15.27	5.24

[a]Self-ratings of sentence comprehension, not scored comprehension as in Experiment 1.

State Test Anxiety and Memory

We conducted a similar set of analyses, using three levels of worry, strategy, and cue on comprehension, free recall, and inference-cued recall separately. The important point to note from these analyses is that level of state test worry was negatively related to comprehension, free recall, and cued recall (significant in all three cases), but did not enter into any interactions with encoding strategy, as did level of depression. Subsequent one-way ANOVAs evaluated state worry effects for free- and cued-recall total scores separately by encoding task condition. In the imagery condition, level of worry was significantly related to both free recall, $F(2, 39) = 5.903, p < .01$, and cued recall, $F(2, 39) = 9.56, p < .001$. In the semantic condition the worry effects were only marginally significant for cued recall ($p < .06$) and not significant for free recall.

Effect Size Comparison

To evaluate the magnitude of the effects associated with depression and anxiety, omega-squared estimates of variance accounted for (Hays, 1988) were calculated and are shown in Figure 1. The depression relations in the imagery condition, shown at the far left of Figure 1, clearly show that the depression effects were nonexistent for cued recall. Conversely, depression accounted for 13.2% of the variance in cued-recall scores in the semantic condition.

Comparatively, the worry effect sizes were clearly of higher magnitude in the imagery condition for cued recall (28.9%), compared with the semantic condition where worry effects accounted for only 9.2% of the cued-recall score variance.

Depression and Anxiety

As with Experiment 1, we examined the interrelations of depression and anxiety measures separately by encoding condition. In the imagery condition, BDI depression scores were significantly correlated with state test worry ($r = .33, p < .05$), but not with emotionality ($r = .21$). In the semantic condition, a pattern similar to but weaker than that observed in Experiment 1 was noted (BDI worry—$r = .54, p < .01$; BDI emotionality—$r = .21$). Thus, in both experiments, the correlation of worry with depression was higher or more positive in the semantic condition than in the imagery condition.

Summary

The results of Experiment 2 produced several interesting effects involving effort toward comprehension. However, in the present context, two points are important. First, we found that depression has effects on memory, and that the effects appear to depend on the encoding task condition. The effect was clearly negative in the semantic condition, but was nonexistent in the imagery condition. This pattern was in partial agreement with Experiment 1, which showed a positive depression–memory correlation in the imagery condition and a negative correlation in the semantic condition. Thus, our two studies suggest that an imagery condition interacts with level of depression to reverse or attenuate the negative effects in some fashion. We speculate on this notion directly.

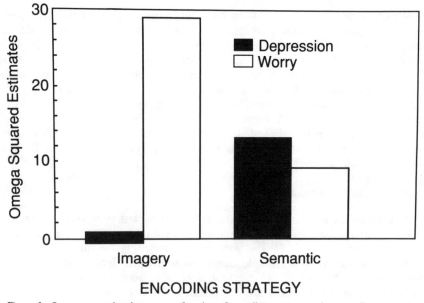

Figure 1   Omega-squared estimates as a function of encoding strategy and personality.

Second, the state test anxiety findings were again consistent with Experiment 1 and our prior studies with this or a similar paradigm. Generally, state test anxiety, primarily the worry component, was negatively related to comprehension, free recall, and cued recall and did not appear to enter into significant interactions with encoding strategy. If anything, the state-anxiety effects appeared stronger in the imagery encoding condition, compared with depression effects, which appeared stronger in the semantic condition. Relatively speaking, state-anxiety effects appeared somewhat stronger than depression effects, although certain methodological issues, which we discuss in the General Discussion, temper our enthusiasm for this effect size difference.

GENERAL DISCUSSION

The primary questions in our two experiments addressed whether the effects of depression on comprehension and sentence memory were mediated by comprehension, and whether the relations would vary as a function of encoding strategy used (imagery or semantic). Additional questions concerned the uniformity of anxiety and depression effects using this sentence memory paradigm and the replicability of the test anxiety findings with our prior research.

Depression-Related Effects

With regard to the viability of the comprehension mediation hypothesis for depression, the present studies are generally negative. The correlation of depression with our direct measure of comprehension was not significant in either encoding condition in Experiment 1, and it was not related to the self-ratings of comprehension in Experiment 2. However, it might be premature to reject the comprehension mediation hypothesis, as the strongest correlations between depression and memory were noted in the inference-cue test; our direct measure of scored comprehension was most strongly related here as well. The comprehension link also varied in direction (positive in the imagery condition and negative in the semantic condition), corresponding to the free-recall and inference-cue correlations. The self-ratings of comprehension in Experiment 2 were unrelated to depression, but they did not themselves correlate with memory performance.

Does the encoding strategy used make a difference? Depression effects were found to be positive with imagery encoding in Experiment 1 and simply nonexistent with imagery encoding in Experiment 2. The effects of depression were negative in the semantic conditions of both experiments. The negative depression effects in the semantic encoding conditions converge with prior evidence that depression effects can be found by using an individual difference approach (as opposed to a mood-induction procedure), a point of recent controversy. In three recent studies, Hasher et al. (1985) failed to find any depression effects on story recall when the BDI was used to classify college students according to level of depression. Ellis (1985) attributed this failure to find depression effects to a combination of a mild mood manipulation (use of the BDI) associated with the use of a task procedure that placed minimal demands on cognitive resources. We found depression effects using the BDI, and the effects varied as a function of encoding strategy, both of which required cognitive effort. We, therefore, agree with Ellis

(1985) about the importance of task characteristics in the study of depression and cognition, but disagree with him on two issues—one methodological, the other more substantive.

Methodologically, it is possible to find reliable depression effects on comprehension and memory using an individual difference approach. In two experiments, using sentence-memory materials, we have shown reliable depression effects by using the BDI to classify students in terms of level of depression. Thus, task characteristics are probably the more important variable when using the BDI. For example, it is possible that Hasher et al.'s (1985) story materials are rich in imagery-evocation potential. If this were the case, collectively we would have five experiments, three by Hasher et al. and the two reported herein that do not find negative depression effects under conditions that evoke imagery.

More substantively, our failure to find negative depression effects under imagery encoding conditions seems inconsistent with Ellis's (1985) views. Because it is not at all clear that imagery is less (or more) effortful than other strategies, the absence of depression effects with imagery encoding is something of a puzzle. Perhaps a motivational explanation should be considered a possibility. Kahneman (1973) pointed out that attentional problems can be of two types. In one case, a person attends to X instead of Y, that is, his or her attention is diverted and performance suffers. In a second type of case, the person has an arousal problem in that he or she does not muster sufficient resources for the task at hand. Beck (1967), for example, considered insufficient motivation to be a central feature of depression. Perhaps depressed persons suffer this latter problem, and under some conditions an imagery task might evoke more arousal and cognitive resources from them. The lack of significant differences related to level of depression and writing speed in Experiment 2, a motivational measure used in depression experiments, is not consistent with this interpretation.

Alternatively, the correlations between depression and worry suggest that imagery may serve to attenuate or eliminate cognitive worry that might distract the depressed person. In the imagery condition of Experiment 1, the correlation between depression and worry was negative, although not significant. The depression–worry correlation, although significant in the imagery condition of Experiment 2, was nonetheless lower in magnitude ($r = .33$) compared with that observed in the semantic condition ($r = .54$). Collectively then, the relation of depression to worry was either nonexistent (Experiment 1) or low in magnitude in the imagery condition (Experiment 2). In contrast, across both experiments the correlation between depression and worry was positive and significant in the semantic encoding condition. Here, higher levels of depression were associated with higher levels of cognitive worry. Thus, it is plausible that the imagery condition served to make the depressed students less worried. The fact that depression–memory correlations were reduced in magnitude when worry was partialed out is supportive of this interpretation. As worry is generally viewed as having a distracting effect on task performance, these data are consistent with a cognitive interference hypothesis of the depression effect (Miller, 1975) as opposed to strictly a motivational account.

The positive relation between depression and memory performance in the imagery condition in Experiment 1 demands more research. It is clearly not typical of previous findings in the depression area; it does not appear to be explainable from either a resource allocation model or a schema theory model of mood effects; and it is not expected from cognitive theories of depression relating depressed mood states to cognitive functioning (e.g., Beck, 1967). The positive finding did not replicate in Experiment 2, however, where no depression effects were noted in the imagery encoding condition. Future research should address this issue.

Anxiety-Related Effects

Compared with the depression effects addressed in these two studies, the test anxiety effects appear to be more straightforward. In our previous studies with the sentence-memory paradigm, we have consistently noted main effects for level of test anxiety, particularly the worry component. The observed worry effects were quite consistent and appeared to hold across a variety of encoding and test conditions, but occasionally they appeared to be moderated by encoding strategy (see Hedl & Bartlett, 1981). On the other hand, emotionality was generally unrelated to memory performance. Where significant emotionality–performance correlations were found, they generally became nonsignificant when the common variance with worry was partialed out. Recent reviews of the test anxiety literature have noted this pattern as well (Deffenbacher, 1980; Morris, Davis, & Hutchings, 1981).

Although comprehension mediation is not supported for depression effects, there is some evidence that it is valid for test anxiety. Hedl and Bartlett (1981, 1982, 1989) have shown that worry is significantly related to sentence comprehension scores as derived in the present experiment (although the correlations were modest). Although this worry–comprehension relation was not significant in Experiment 1, the pattern of worry–cued recall correlations is supportive of a comprehension mediation hypothesis. Similar to the depression findings, the test anxiety correlations were strong in the inference-cue test for both encoding task conditions. Also, the comprehension–recall correlations were more robust in the inference-cue test condition as well. More important, the multiple regression analyses of Experiment 1 demonstrated that worry effects were attenuated when comprehension was included in the model. In contrast, depression remained a reliable predictor of memory performance with similar analytic methodology.

In summary, the present study examined depression, anxiety, and comprehension effects in sentence memory. A number of parallels to the research literature were noted. The test anxiety data were generally consistent with our prior studies that used this paradigm and with the more general test anxiety literature. The similarity of test anxiety effects across the two encoding task conditions suggests a quantitative effect for the emotional state of anxiety. That is, anxiety is interfering with a memory process that underlies performance in a variety of task conditions.

The depression effects, however, were inconsistent and depended on the nature of the encoding task and task materials. This pattern is suggestive of a qualitative effect. That is, different processes were affected by the two encoding strategies, and the result varied by level of depression and sentence materials. It was not possible to isolate the mechanism(s) responsible for the different depression effects, but a case was made for the role of cognitive worry.

A few cautions are in order, particularly concerning the interpretation of any differences between depression and anxiety effects on memory. The present experiments involved a correlational approach and did not involve an experimental manipulation of mood state. Only encoding strategy was varied between subjects.

The depression and anxiety scores were obtained from the same subjects, and the order of data collection was varied. The depression scores were obtained before the experiments and the anxiety scores were obtained after each experiment, using retrospective state instructions to infer the presence of test anxiety during the experiment. Thus, it is problematic to compare depression and anxiety effects directly, given these methodological differences.

It will remain for future work to compare the effects of test anxiety and depression as discrete emotional states on learning, memory, and cognition, using some type of between-subjects manipulation of mood. It is, of course, difficult to develop manipulations of pure mood state (Polivy, 1981), but such manipulations, if successful, would be crucial for studying the comparative effects of these different emotional states. The continued investigation of the attenuating effects of imagery with depressed subjects would seem to be a fruitful endeavor.

REFERENCES

Auble, P. M., & Franks, J. J. (1978). The effects of effort toward comprehension on recall. *Memory and Cognition, 6*, 20–25.

Auble, P. M., Franks, J. J., & Soraci, S. A., Jr. (1979). Effort toward comprehension: Elaboration of "aha!"? *Memory and Cognition, 7*, 426–434.

Beck, A. T. (1967). *Depression: Clinical, experimental, and theoretical aspects.* New York: Harper & Row.

Beck, A. T., Ward, C. H., Mendelson, M., Mock, J., & Erbaugh, J. (1961). An inventory for measuring depression. *Archives of General Psychiatry, 4*, 561–571.

Bower, G. H. (1981). Mood and memory. *American Psychologist, 36*, 129–148.

Bumberry, W., Oliver, J. M., & McClure, J. N. (1978). Validation of the Beck Depression Inventory on a university population using psychiatric estimate as the criterion. *Journal of Experimental Psychology: General, 1*, 268–294.

Craik, F. I. M., & Tulving, E. (1975). Depth of processing and the retention of words in episodic memory. *Journal of Experimental Psychology: General, 1*, 268–294.

Deffenbacher, J. L. (1980). Worry and emotionality in test anxiety. In I. G. Sarason (Ed.), *Test anxiety: Theory, research, and applications* (pp. 111–128). Hillsdale, NJ: Erlbaum.

Edmunsen, E. D., & Nelson, D. L. (1976). Anxiety, imagery, and sensory interference. *Bulletin of the Psychonomic Society, 8*, 319–322.

Ellis, H. C. (1985). On the importance of mood intensity and encoding demands in memory: Commentary on Hasher, Rose, Zacks, Sanft, and Doren. *Journal of Experimental Psychology: General, 114*, 392–395.

Ellis, H. C., Thomas, R. L., McFarland, A. D., & Lane, J. W. (1985). Emotional mood states and retrieval in episodic memory. *Journal of Experimental Psychology: Learning, Memory, and Cognition, 11*, 363–370.

Ellis, H. C., Thomas, R. L., & Rodriquez, I. A. (1984). Emotional mood states and memory: Elaborative encoding, semantic processing, and cognitive effort. *Journal of Experimental Psychology: General, 10*, 470–482.

Eysenck, M. W. (1982). *Attention, and arousal: Cognition and performance.* Berlin, Federal Republic of Germany: Springer-Verlag.

Hasher, L., & Zacks, R. T. (1979). Automatic and effortful processes in memory. *Journal of Experimental Psychology: General, 108*, 336–388.

Hasher, L., Rose, K. C., Zacks, R. T., Sanft, H., & Doren, B. (1985). Mood, recall, and selectivity effects in normal college students. *Journal of Experimental Psychology: General, 114*, 104–118.

Hays, W. L. (1988). *Statistics* (4th ed.). New York: Holt, Rinehart & Winston.

Hedl, J. J., Jr., & Bartlett, J. C. (1981, April). *Test anxiety and sentence memory.* Paper presented at the meeting of the American Educational Research Association, New York.

Hedl, J. J., Jr., & Bartlett, J. C. (1982, March). *Toward improving the magnitude of test anxiety and sentence memory relationships.* Paper presented at the meeting of the American Education Research Association, New York.

Hedl, J. J., Jr., & Bartlett, J. C. (1985, March). *Test anxiety and effort-toward-comprehension in sentence memory.* Paper presented at the meeting of the American Education Research Association, Chicago.

Hedl, J. J., Jr., & Bartlett, J. C. (1989). Test anxiety, sentence comprehension, and recognition memory. *Anxiety Research: An International Journal, 1,* 269–279.

Johnson, M. K., Bransford, J. D., & Soloman, S. (1973). Memory for tacit implications of sentences. *Journal of Experimental Psychology, 98,* 203–205.

Kahneman, D. (1973). *Attention and effort.* Englewood Cliffs, NJ: Prentice-Hall.

Krohne, H. W., & Laux, L. (Eds.). (1982). *Achievement, stress, and anxiety.* Washington, DC: Hemisphere.

Leight, K. A., & Ellis, H. C. (1981). Emotional mood states, strategies, and state-dependency in memory. *Journal of Verbal Learning and Verbal Behavior, 20,* 257–266.

Levin, J. R. (1981). On functions of pictures in prose. In F. J. Pirozzolo & M. C. Wittrock (Eds.), *Neuropsychological and cognitive processes in reading* (pp. 203–228). New York: Academic Press.

Miller, W. R. (1975). Psychological deficit in depression. *Psychological Bulletin, 82,* 238–260.

Morris, L. W., Davis, M. A., & Hutchings, C. A. (1981). Cognitive and emotional components of anxiety: Literature review and a revised worry-emotionality scale. *Journal of Educational Psychology, 73,* 541–555.

O'Neil, H. F., Jr. (1978). *Learning strategies.* New York: Academic Press.

O'Neil, H. F., Jr., & Spielberger, C. D. (Eds.). (1979). *Cognitive and affective learning strategies.* New York: Academic Press.

Paivio, A., & Descrochers, A. (1981). Mnemonic techniques in second-language learning. *Journal of Educational Psychology, 73,* 780–795.

Peters, E. E., Levin, J. R., McGivern, J. E., & Pressley, M. (1985). Further comparison of representational and transformation prose-learning imagery. *Journal of Educational Psychology, 77,* 129–136.

Polivy, J. (1981). On the induction of emotion in the laboratory: Discrete moods or multiple affect states. *Journal of Personality and Social Psychology, 41,* 803–817.

Pressley, M., Symons, S., McDaniel, M. A., Snyder, B. L., & Turnure, J. E. (1988). Elaborative interrogation facilitates acquisition of confusing facts. *Journal of Educational Psychology, 80,* 268–278.

Sarason, I. G. (1980). *Test anxiety: Theory, research, and applications.* Hillsdale, NJ: Erlbaum.

Schultz, K. D. (1978). Imagery and the control of depression. In J. L. Singer & K. S. Pope (Eds.), *The power of human imagination: New methods in psychotherapy* (pp. 281–307). New York: Plenum Press.

Schwarzer, R., Jerusalem, M., & Schwarzer, C. (1983). Self-related and situation-related cognitions in test anxiety: A longitudinal analysis with structural equations. In H. M. van der Ploeg, R. Schwarzer, & C. D. Spielberger (Eds.), *Advances in test anxiety research* (Vol. 2, pp. 35–43). Lisse, the Netherlands: Swets & Zeitlinger.

Schwarzer, R., Jerusalem, M., & Stiksrud, A. (1984). The developmental relationship between test anxiety and helplessness. In H. M. van der Ploeg, R. Schwarzer, & C. D. Spielberger (Eds.) *Advances in test anxiety research* (Vol. 3, pp. 73–79). Lisse, the Netherlands: Swets & Zeitlinger.

Schwarzer, R., van der Ploeg, H. M., & Spielberger, C. D. (Eds.). (1982). *Advances in test anxiety research* (Vol. 1). Hillsdale, NJ: Erlbaum.

Schwarzer, R., van der Ploeg, H. M., & Spielberger, C. D. (Eds.). (1987). *Advances in test anxiety research* (Vol. 5). Hillsdale, NJ: Erlbaum.

Sheikh, A. A., & Sheikh, K. S. (1985). *Imagery in education.* Farmingdale, NY: Baywood.

Spielberger, C. D. (1980). *Preliminary manual for the Test Anxiety Inventory.* Palo Alto, CA: Consulting Psychologists Press.

Till, R. E. (1977). Sentence memory prompted with inferential recall cues. *Journal of Experimental Psychology: Human Learning and Memory, 3,* 129–141.

Till, R. E. (1985). Verbatim and inferential memory in young and elderly subjects. *Journal of Gerontology, 40,* 316–323.

Till, R. E., Cormak, D. R., & Prince, P. L. (1977). Effects of orienting tasks on sentence comprehension and cued recall. *Memory and Cognition, 5,* 59–66.

Till, R. E., & Walsh, D. A. (1980). Encoding and retrieval factors in adult memory for implicational sentences. *Journal of Verbal Learning and Verbal Behavior, 19,* 1–16.

Van der Ploeg, H. M., Schwarzer, R., & Spielberger, C. D. (Eds.). (1983–1985). *Advances in test anxiety research.* (Vols. 2–4). Hillsdale, NJ: Erlbaum.

Weinstein, C. E., Underwood, V. L., Wicker, F. W., & Cubberly, W. R. (1979). Cognitive learning strategies: Verbal and imaginal elaboration. In H. F. O'Neil, Jr., & C. D. Spielberger (Eds.), *Cognitive and affective learning strategies* (pp. 45–75). New York: Academic Press.

9

Importance of Outcome as a Determinant of Anxiety

Peter Schulz
University of Trier, Federal Republic of Germany

In research on test anxiety, a distinction is made between the cognitive and motivational components of anxiety. Liebert and Morris (1967) labeled these two components *worry* and *emotionality* and constructed state measures of them. The conceptual distinction between worry and emotionality has proved useful in test anxiety research (Schwarzer, 1981; Wine, 1971) and has stimulated the development of measures of these constructs as components of test anxiety as a situational-specific personality trait (Spielberger, 1980; Spielberger, Gonzalez, Taylor, Algaze, & Anton, 1978).

Emotionality is generally regarded as the motivational component of test anxiety. This construct refers to feeling states of uneasiness, tension, and nervousness and concomitant changes in the level of physiological functioning that are experienced in examination situations. Worry, on the other hand, is conceptualized as the cognitive component of anxiety. This construct involves negative task expectations, self-evaluations, and concern about one's level of performance (Eysenck, 1979; Liebert & Morris, 1967; Sarason, 1975). Failure feedback typically affects the worry component of anxiety more than the emotionality component (Morris & Liebert, 1973).

This chapter deals primarily with emotionality and the factors that influence this component of test anxiety. In an effort to clarify this concept, the importance of behavioral outcomes is analyzed as one of the primary determinants of emotionality. The position taken here is that subjects whose motivation for coping with the task is low will not be emotionally aroused and hence will begin to deflect to another task when task difficulty increases (Schulz & Schönpflug, 1982). On the contrary, subjects whose need to cope with the tasks is high cannot deflect when confronted with difficult tasks. Thus, whether a discrepancy between demand and capacity leads to anxiety depends on outcome importance.

Importance of outcome results from the subjective significance of an activity-outcome relation (Heckhausen, 1980; Schwarzer, 1981; Wortman & Brehm, 1975). If an outcome of a subject's activity has no significance, a lack of control has no or few emotional consequences (Dweck & Wortman, 1982; Schwarzer, 1981). Only an outcome that is important for the subject can affect self-esteem. This integration of valence and competence aspects in the definition of anxiety is neglected in anxiety research (Hackfort, 1983).

The experimental study reported in this chapter was conducted to test the hypothesis that importance of outcome is the main condition of the occurrence of emotionality as a component of anxiety.

METHOD

The Experimental Design

The Experimental Group

To induce a high level of outcome importance, 2 subjects had to solve a common task together. Subject A, who collaborated with the experimenter, was given a slide with a so-called total task, simulating features of clerical work. This task contained a subtask, which had to be solved by the other subject, B, before Subject A could solve the common task. Subject B had to solve the subtask within a time limit of 50 s. This period was called the "period of information processing" (Table 1).

After 50 s, the task presentation was terminated automatically, and Subject B was instructed to communicate the solution to Subject A. As can be seen in Table 1, this period was called the "period of responding." The solution was communicated via a digital counter that could be seen by both subjects. With the solution to the subtask, Subject A could then complete the total task, again within a 50-s time limit. Meanwhile, Subject B had to wait for feedback as to whether his or her solution was correct or not. This period was called the "period of waiting." After Subject A had also communicated the task's solution, both subjects received feedback. Only the joint result, if it was correct, was rewarded with money. Both subjects received deutsche marks (DM) 1 for a correct solution. If the task solution was incorrect, DM 1 was subtracted from a pool of money (DM 30) the subjects received for joining the experiment. This period was called the "period of feedback." A digital counter displayed the common premium. When the joint task solution was wrong, the subjects were informed as to who had made the mistake.

The Control Group

To induce a low level of outcome importance, a control group, consisting of an equal number of pairs, worked at the same tasks in the same order; however, a joint solution was not demanded and feedback was not provided (no-feedback period).

Eighteen pairs of subjects were tested within each group. However, only the reactions of Subject B were analyzed because Subject A was a confederate of the experimenter and was familiar with the tasks. The subjects—students of the Uni-

Table 1 The Activity Periods During Experimental Work

Periods	Activity	Time limits (s)
1. Information processing	The subject works at the subtask.	50
2. Responding	The subject communicates the task solution to his or her coworker.	20
3. Waiting	The subject waits until his or her coworker has finished.	50
4. Feedback	The subjects receive feedback on their outcome.	20

versity of Trier—were recruited through an announcement. The sample consisted of 24 men and 12 women. The mean age was 26. The total experimental work was arranged in two blocks of 10 tasks. Thus, all 36 pairs of subjects had to solve 20 tasks, with a 3-min break after 10 tasks. In addition to these two "periods of recovery," a third recovery period was given before the experimental work and before the subjects were instructed. Thus, there were three periods of recovery: before, during, and after the experimental work.

To obtain homogeneous groups in regard to the demand/capacity ratio, we measured subjects' intelligence (Amthauer, 1953) before the experiment and assigned them to groups according to their intelligence scores.

Dependent Variables

During the various activity periods, simultaneous recordings of three cardiovascular responses were taken continuously: heart rate, pulse transit time, and finger pulse amplitude. These cardiovascular responses were recorded by means of a cardiovascular monitor system based on a Z-80 microprocessor. In recording heart rate, the cardiac signal was converted to a step function measure of heart rate. Pulse wave velocity was measured by monitoring the time interval between the R-wave of the electrocardiogram and the maximum of radial pressure pulse. The resulting pulse transit time, measured in milliseconds, is suitable for use as an indirect measure of blood pressure changes (Steptoe, Smulyan, & Gribbin, 1976). The higher the pulse transit time, the lower the mean blood pressure, and vice versa. The finger pulse amplitude was measured by recording the changes of peripheral blood volume in arbitrary units. The signal was obtained via a photoelectric transducer placed on the middle finger of the left hand.

In addition to these cardiovascular responses, we asked subjects for introspective reports concerning the experience of stress during the experimental work and we measured state anxiety (using the State–Trait Anxiety Inventory, or STAI; Spielberger, Goruch, & Lushene, 1970; German version by Laux, Glanzman, Schaffner, & Spielberger, 1981) before and after the experiment. Moreover, the number of errors was counted.

RESULTS

Behavioral Data

The only behavioral data gathered in this study were the number of errors. The mean error rate of the experimental group was 0.58; that of the control group was 0.54. Examination of the univariate analysis of variance (ANOVA) for error rate revealed no significant effect between the groups, $F(1, 32) = 0.53$, ns.

Introspective Data

Because state anxiety was measured twice—before and after the experiment—it was possible to evaluate the treatment effect on changes in anxiety scores (Table 2).

As can be seen from Table 2, during experimental work state anxiety increased

Table 2 Changes of State Anxiety and Emotionality During Experimental Work

Measures of state anxiety	Importance of outcome		F	p
	High	Low		
Complete items of the STAI				
Before	39.7	40.7	0.15	ns
After	41.1	36.3	4.63	0.05
Difference	1.4	−4.2	5.68	0.05
Six items of the STAI indicating emotionality				
Before	9.9	10.2	0.10	ns
After	10.8	8.8	7.38	0.01
Difference	0.9	−1.4	7.61	0.01
Remaining items of the STAI				
Before	28.1	28.6	0.05	ns
After	28.6	26.0	2.12	ns
Difference	0.5	−2.6	2.73	ns

Note. STAI = State–Trait Anxiety Inventory.

in the experimental group and decreased in the control group. Table 2 also shows that only the emotionality component of state anxiety was affected by the treatment condition. A univariate ANOVA based on the sum of all item scores measuring emotionality (according to Laux et al., 1981, six items said to measure emotionality were selected) revealed significant group effects for emotionality measured after the experiment and for the difference scores of emotionality. The analysis of the baseline emotionality values revealed no significant effect between the groups. The sum of the remaining item scores yielded no significant difference before or after the experiment. In sum, Table 2 indicates that only the emotionality component of anxiety was affected by treatment condition.

As mentioned earlier, the concomitant feeling states of state anxiety can be described "as consisting of unpleasant, consciously-perceived feelings of tension and apprehension" (Spielberger, 1972, p. 29). Table 3 contains some results of the postexperimental questionnaire concerning those feelings.

The values, as presented in Table 3, represent the group mean of answers from

Table 3 Results of the Postexperimental Questionnaire Concerning the Feeling States of Anxiety Determined by the Experimental Work

Item content	Importance of outcome		F	p
	High	Low		
How did the total stress of the experiment affect your feelings?				
I got nervous	2.44	1.83	7.64	0.01
I got impatient	2.11	1.50	8.54	0.01
I got out of humor	2.06	1.22	9.44	0.01
I got feelings of tension	2.83	2.67	0.35	ns
I was unable to concentrate	2.50	2.22	1.15	ns
I got helpless	1.39	1.44	0.08	ns
I got dissatisfied	2.06	1.83	1.00	ns

a four-level rating scale. We asked for an answer to the question, "How does the total stress of the experiment affect your feelings?" As can be seen from Table 3, subjects in the experimental group became more nervous and more impatient during experimental work. They also became out of humor as compared with the control group. There were no differences, however, in concentration, helplessness, and dissatisfaction. Moreover, no more feelings of tension were recorded in this group.

Emotionality manifests itself not only in feelings of tension and nervousness, but also changes of physiological functioning, including the perception of those changes. Therefore, after the experiment was finished, we asked for an answer to the following statement: "In the recovery periods I was disturbed by perceiving my bodily reactions." The group mean of answers from a four-level rating scale differed between the groups (experimental group, $M = 2.44$; control group, $M = 1.74$). The ANOVA yielded a significant group effect, $F(1, 32) = 7.74, p < 0.01$. This result indicates that the subjects of the experimental group were more disturbed by the perception of their bodily reactions, particularly in resting periods.

Physiological Data

To reduce the physiological data, the mean response level for each activity period was calculated (see Table 1 for various activity periods). Thus, for each activity period three cardiovascular parameters were obtained:

1. Heart rate level—Heart rate (HR) in beats per minute averaged over the first 10 tasks (Block 1) and the second 10 tasks (Block 2).
2. Level of pulse transit time—Pulse transit time (PTT) in milliseconds averaged over Block 1 and Block 2.
3. Level of finger pulse amplitude—Finger pulse amplitude (FPA) in arbitrary units averaged over Block 1 and Block 2.

The following analysis of the cardiovascular responses is based on the activity structure illustrated in Table 1. We analyzed the changes of response level from one activity period to the other. According to the experimental procedure, the work began with the presentation of the task. The subjects had to process information and then communicate the solution of the task to their coworker. Therefore, we begin the analysis of the physiological data with the changes in cardiovascular response level from the period of information processing to the period of responding (Table 4).

As can be seen in Table 4, HR increases from information processing to responding when outcome is important and decreases when outcome is not important. An ANOVA based on difference scores was computed and yielded high significant effects between the groups for both blocks. The treatment effect on changes in PTT was rather similar to that observed for HR (note that a decrease in PTT reflects an increase in blood pressure). As can be seen in Table 4, the PTT decreases from information processing to responding in the experimental group and increases in the control group. Again the ANOVA, based on difference scores, yielded highly significant group effects for both blocks. The treatment effect on changes in FPA was similar to those for HR and PTT, although the effects were not

Table 4 Changes of Cardiovascular Response Level from the Period of Information Processing to the Period of Responding for Two Blocks of Tasks

Cardiovascular parameter and block	Importance of outcome		F	p
	High	Low		
Heart rate level				
1	2.0	−4.7	18.64	.001
2	1.6	−4.9	33.27	.001
Level of pulse transmit time				
1	−2.0	6.0	25.72	.001
2	−2.0	3.6	17.13	.001
Level of finger pulse amplitude				
1	−9.0	0.56	3.38	.10
2	−3.5	−1.2	1.09	ns

significant. We observed a vasoconstriction reaction from information processing to responding only in the experimental group.

After communicating the solution, the subject had to wait until the coworker had finished his or her work. Therefore, we next analyzed the changes in response level from the period of responding to the period of waiting (Table 5).

As can be seen from Table 5, in the experimental group we observed a significantly greater decrease in HR from the responding period to the waiting period. However, the increase in PTT was similar for the two groups. The FPA level shows a further vasoconstriction reaction from responding to waiting, although the group differences failed to reach statistical significance.

According to the activity structure (Table 1), the changes of the physiological response from the period of waiting to the feedback period should be analyzed. However, because feedback was only provided for the experimental group, Table 6 shows changes in response level from the period of waiting to the period of information processing.

As can be seen in Table 6, HR increases from the waiting period to the information-processing period. There is no difference between the groups. In line

Table 5 Changes of Cardiovascular Response Level from the Period of Responding to the Period of Waiting for Two Blocks of Tasks

Cardiovascular parameter and block	Importance of outcome		F	p
	High	Low		
Heart rate level				
1	−7.3	−1.1	27.20	0.01
2	−5.2	−0.2	15.78	0.01
Level of pulse transmit time				
1	5.2	3.2	1.60	ns
2	4.2	1.8	3.16	ns
Level of finger pulse amplitude				
1	−1.3	4.5	2.80	ns
2	−5.1	0.8	3.35	0.10

Table 6 Changes of Cardiovascular Response Level from the Period of Waiting to the Period of Information Processing for Two Blocks of Tasks

Cardiovascular parameter and block	Importance of outcome		F	p
	High	Low		
Heart rate level				
1	5.4	5.7	0.04	*ns*
2	3.5	5.0	0.82	*ns*
Level of pulse transmit time				
1	−3.4	−9.2	7.32	.01
2	−2.2	−5.2	3.12	*ns*
Level of finger pulse amplitude				
1	−10.3	5.1	8.18	.01
2	−8.5	−0.4	4.04	.05

with the HR increase, PTT decreased for both groups, but the control group showed higher scores. This treatment effect is significant only in Block 1. The analysis of FPA changes revealed a different pattern. The ANOVA for the period of information processing as a change from the waiting period yielded a significant treatment effect for both blocks of tasks (Table 6). We observed a distinct vasoconstriction reaction in the period of information processing as a change from waiting period only in the experimental group.

Besides the analysis of changes in response level from one activity period to the other, we also analyzed the course of cardiovascular responses over the three recovery periods. Physiological activity was recorded during three recovery periods: (a) before the experimental work (and before the tasks were explained to the subjects); (b) during experimental work, (e.g., in between the two blocks of tasks); and (c) after the experiment was finished. During these periods, subjects were instructed to relax for 3 min. A 2 × 3 factorial ANOVA with repeated measures (three recovery periods) on the last factor for all three physiological parameters revealed no Treatment × Period interaction. Thus, the experimental manipulation had no influence on changes of the cardiovascular response level from one recovery period to the other.

In addition to response level, we also calculated the response variability for the three recovery periods. The variability scores were obtained by computing the standard deviation of each of the cardiovascular parameters. The standard deviation score was calculated from second-by-second recordings over the 3 min of each recovery period.

Figure 1 shows the HR variability during the three recovery periods. The effects of the treatment condition on the variability scores were explored by performing a one-way ANOVA computed for each period separately. The HR variability during the initial recovery period did not differ between the groups, $F(1, 32) = 0.35$, *ns*. However, during the recovery period between the two blocks of tasks, the ANOVA yielded a significant treatment effect, $F(1, 32) = 7.69, p < 0.01$. For the last recovery period the group difference again disappeared, $F(1, 32) = 2.34$, *ns*. This reaction pattern was independent of intelligence.

The PTT variability scores show a reaction pattern similar to that already observed in HR variability (Figure 2).

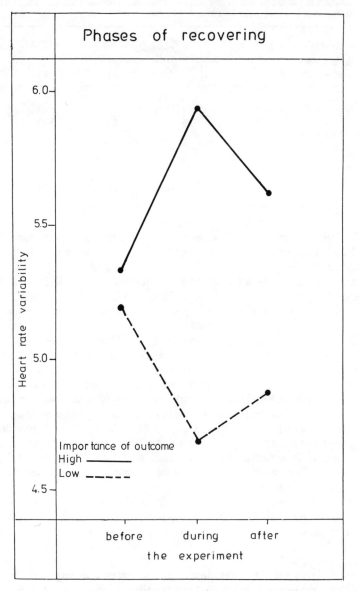

Figure 1 Mean heart rate variability during the three recovery periods.

As Figure 2 illustrates, we found no group difference in PTT variability during the recovery period before the experiment, $F(1, 32) = 0.03$, *ns*. During the other two recovery periods, however, significant group differences were observed; recovery period between the two blocks of tasks, $F(1, 32) = 8.80$, $p < 0.01$; recovery period after the experiment was finished, $F(1, 32) = 4.66$, $p < 0.05$. The differences were mainly due to low-intelligent subjects.

The effect of the experimental condition on FPA variability scores is shown in Figure 3.

As can be seen from Figure 3, the FPA variability scores show a reaction pattern already observed by HR and PTT variability. Although there was no group effect during the recovery period before the experimental work, $F(1, 32) = 2.69$,

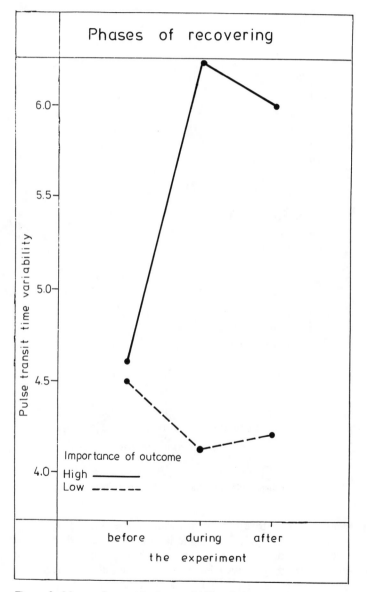

Figure 2 Mean pulse transit time variability during the three recovery periods.

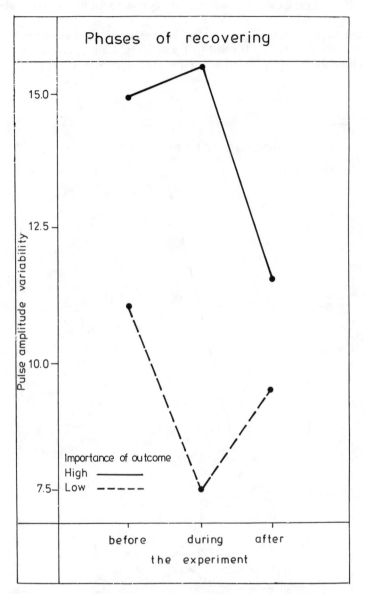

Figure 3 Mean finger pulse amplitude during the three recovery periods.

ns, we again found a treatment effect during the second recovery period, $F(1, 32) = 16.91$, $p < 0.01$. During the last recovery period, the group difference again disappeared, $F(1, 32) = 0.64$, *ns.* The group difference during the second recovery period again was due to the low-intelligent subjects.

The reaction pattern of the HR, PTT, and FPA variability scores over the three recovery periods can be summarized as follows: During the recovery period before the experiment, there were no group differences observed. In contrast, during the recovery period in between the two parts of the experimental work all three variability scores yielded highly significant group differences, whereas during the third recovery period, after finishing experimental work, only the PTT variability scores differed between the groups.

DISCUSSION

The main assumption tested in this experiment was the hypothesis that it is the emotionality component of anxiety rather than the worry component that is affected by different levels of outcome importance (e.g., that importance of outcome is the main condition for the occurrence of emotionality). The question of whether the present results support this hypothesis arises.

The evidence of recent research in test anxiety indicates that emotionality bears no consistent relation to performance (Morris & Liebert, 1973; Schwarzer, 1981; Wine, 1971). Hence, we expected no differences in performance between the groups. This prediction was confirmed by the error rate. As a result of our experiment, we found no differences in error rate, whether outcome was important or not, although the analysis of error rate indicates that the task difficulty in combination with the time pressure was suitable to impose a task demand that slightly outbalanced capacity.

The main evidence supporting our hypothesis, however, comes from the introspective data (Tables 2 and 3). The results concerning the changes in state anxiety suggest that importance of outcome primarily affects the emotionality component of anxiety. Although we found a high error rate and thus expected an increase in worry, only the emotionality scores revealed significant group differences. Following Laux et al. (1981), the remaining items of the STAI cannot be definitely assigned to either worry or emotionality. So it seems apparent that the group difference, observed also in the remaining items of Table 2, is definitely not due to differences in worry. All together, the component analysis of state anxiety changes seems to support our hypothesis. Nevertheless, it is necessary to reproduce our findings with a test anxiety inventory that better separates the emotionality and worry components of anxiety.

Aside from this component analysis of state anxiety changes, our hypothesis is further confirmed by the results presented in Table 3. These data show that if outcome is important, subjects became nervous, impatient, and out of humor, but did not rate themselves as more unable to concentrate, helpless, or dissatisfied during the experiment. Contrary to Eysenck (1979), who postulated that emotionality—among others—involves a state of tension, our results seem to indicate that emotionality involves no negative feeling states or aversive perceived emotions. According to our results, emotionality involves an unspecific feeling state, which is better characterized in terms of nervousness, impatience, and getting out of humor.

The results concerning changes of cardiovascular responses from the period of information processing to the responding period (Table 4) demonstrate that we succeeded in manipulating the importance of outcome. We observed a cardiac acceleration in the period of responding, when outcome is important, whereas we found a deceleration when it was not important. This was indicated by HR changes as well as by PTT changes. Even the FPA changes support this interpretation, although the group differences failed to reach statistical significance. It seems that the sympathetically mediated HR and blood pressure increase reflects a greater emotional involvement during this period. That means that the subjects were more emotionally involved while communicating the result to a coworker, although only when the result was of significance for the coworker.

Although the cardiovascular responses of the experimental group show a further cardiac acceleration next to the information-processing period, before returning to the waiting baseline and immediately following information processing, the control group returned to the baseline level of the waiting period (see Tables 4 and 5). The greater decrease in HR and increase in PTT of the experimental group (Table 5) seems to compensate the foregoing further cardiac acceleration. This interpretation is supported by a result not mentioned earlier: During the waiting period all three cardiovascular response levels did not differ between the groups (e.g., all subjects had identical baselines).

The examination of cardiovascular responses during information processing as changed from the period of waiting revealed still another interesting result. Besides an HR acceleration and a blood pressure increase, an additional vasoconstriction reaction occurred during information processing, but only when outcome was important to the subjects. If there was no need for a perfect solution, a peripheral vasoconstriction during this period was not observed (Table 6). A possible explanation for this finding is that the additional vasoconstriction reaction occurred because there was a great incentive for effortful coping with the tasks at hand—the outcome was important (e.g., the subjects had an enhanced need to reach a perfect solution and thus had a greater effort expenditure when working on the tasks). This need to exert control was accompanied by an increased number of cardiovascular regulatory mechanisms involved.

Besides the further cardiac acceleration during responding and the additional vasoconstriction during information processing, we observed a further treatment effect: a higher labilization of all three cardiovascular parameters during the recovery period between the two parts of the experimental work. This period was characterized by the following features: (a) The subjects already had experience with the difficult tasks and had already made mistakes, and (b) the subjects knew they had to solve further tasks of the same level of difficulty with the same probability of failure. In our view, this was a real-life situation. Thus, our data indicate that a labilization of cardiovascular response in this typical daily life situation occurs when the outcome is important for the subjects and the probability of failure is high. The more mistakes that are made, the greater the labilization. The fact that the subjects with lower intelligence scores had higher labilization scores supports this conclusion.

According to Schönpflug (1983), subjects are free to engage in various activities during the recovery periods. Subjects are given an opportunity to orientate themselves with the forthcoming demands and with their own persons. During the recovery period between the experimental task blocks, the subject could think about how well he or she had coped with the preceding tasks, and how well he or she might cope with the forthcoming tasks (see also Otto, 1982; Wieland & Schönpflug, 1980). So it seems that the higher labilization scores were due to more involvement in preparation and orientation.

As our results indicate, subjects perceived the cardiovascular labilization during the recovery period between the two experimental sessions. As reported earlier, the subjects in the experimental group were more disturbed by their bodily reactions, particularly in those activity periods where they did not concentrate on the tasks. As Schönpflug (1983) pointed out, self-regulatory skills are important in waiting situations because there are no external demands calling for immediate attention. The internal sensations of arousal constitute the main demands for regulation.

In summary, the results concerning the physiological correlates of emotionality lead to the following findings:

1. If outcome was important, we observed a further cardiac acceleration in activity periods in which subjects communicated an outcome of their activity to other people.

2. If outcome was important, a vasoconstriction reaction occurred in addition to HR increase and PTT decrease during those periods in which the outcomes were produced.

3. If outcome was important and the demands outbalanced capacity, we found a labilization of cardiovascular responses in the periods between experimental sessions.

These findings have implications for the etiology of coronary heart disease. The risk for hypertension, and thus for coronary heart disease, increases (a) the more frequently high blood pressure increases occur, (b) the more a labilization of the systolic blood pressure is observed, and (c) the more a person reacts with a vasoconstriction reaction to psychological stress (Schaefer & Blohmke, 1977; Schmidt, 1982). If this generalization of our findings is correct, we can conclude that the combination of two factors, outcome importance and demands–capacity imbalance, increases the risk of hypertension.

Before concluding, we should discuss a further aspect of our results. We found that emotionality increased if the outcome became more important. This result allows us to explain why high-anxious subjects (trait anxiety) react with higher levels of state anxiety when confronted with difficult tasks (Spielberger, 1972). According to our findings, it can be assumed that when confronted with a difficult task, the subjects high in trait anxiety react with a higher emotionality because the outcome is generally more important for them.

The question arises as to why outcomes are generally more important for high-anxious subjects, particularly when they are working together with others. A number of experimental studies have indicated that high-anxious persons have the tendency to attribute their failures to internal, stable factors (e.g., their abilities; Kukla, 1972; Schulz & Schönpflug, 1982; Weiner & Potepan, 1970). As these attributions lead to negative self-esteem and thus to negative feelings, the outcome is of higher significance for these subjects. Thus, for these subjects there exists only one opportunity to reduce the threat to their self-esteem: They have to prevent failures, particularly if the outcomes are evaluated by other people (Becker, 1982; Wine, 1982). However, if these subjects are not able to prevent failures, negative feelings and deteriorating effects are a consequence (Kuhl, 1983). Thus, importance of outcome can be viewed as both a motivating factor (if capacity reaches the demand) and a stress factor (if demands outbalance capacity).

SUMMARY

This chapter has dealt with emotionality as a component of test anxiety. An attempt was made to provide a concept in which importance of outcome is analyzed as the primary determinant of emotionality. To test this hypothesis, an experiment was conducted. In the experimental group, 2 subjects solved a common task together. Only the joint result, if correct, was rewarded with money. When the joint task solution was wrong, the subjects were informed as to which of them had made the mistake. A control group worked at the same tasks in the same order, but a joint solution was not demanded. We expected that the treatment condition would increase the importance of the outcome. The 36 pairs of subjects, 18 pairs within each group, had to solve 20 tasks, with a 3-min break after 10 tasks. The dependent variables were overt behavior, physiological activity, and introspective reports. State anxiety was measured before and after the experiment. The results support the hypothesis outlined earlier. It was found that only the emotionality component of anxiety was affected by our treatment condition. The physiological correlates of emotionality and its implications for the etiology of coronary heart disease were discussed.

REFERENCES

Amthauer, R. (1953). *Intelligenz-Struktur-Test. Handanweisung für die Durchführung und Auswertung* [Intelligence-structure-test: Manual for accomplishment and evaluation]. Göttingen, Federal Republic of Germany: Hogrefe.

Becker, P. (1982). Towards a process analysis of test anxiety: Some theoretical and methodological observations. In R. Schwarzer, H. M. van der Ploeg, & C. D. Spielberger (Eds.), *Advances in test anxiety research* (Vol. 1, pp. 11–17). Lisse, the Netherlands: Swets & Zeitlinger.

Dweck, C. S., & Wortman, C. B. (1982). Learned helplessness, anxiety, and achievement motivation. In H. W. Krohne & L. Laux (Eds.), *Achievement, stress, and anxiety* (pp. 93–125). New York: Hemisphere.

Eysenck, M. W. (1979). Anxiety, learning, and memory: A reconceptualization. *Journal of Research in Personality, 13*, 363–385.

Hackfort, D. (1983). *Theorie und Diagnostik sportbezogener Ängstlichkeit* [Theory and diagnostic of sport related anxiety]. Unpublished doctoral dissertation, Cologne, Federal Republic of Germany.

Heckhausen, H. (1980). *Motivation und Handeln* [Motivation and activity]. Berlin, Federal Republic of Germany: Springer.

Kuhl, U. (1983). Aspekte der Leistungsmotivation in der Trainer-Athlet-Beziehung [Aspects of achievement motivation in the relationship between trainer and sportsman]. *Leistungssport, 5*, 51–53.

Kukla, A. (1972). Cognitive determinants of achieving behavior. *Journal of Personality and Social Psychology, 21*, 166–174.

Laux, L., Glanzmann, P., Schaffner, P., & Spielberger, C. D. (1981). *Das State-Trait-Angstinventar. Theoretische Grundlagen und Handlungsanweisung* [The state-trait-anxiety inventory. Theoretical foundations and manual]. Weinheim: Beltz.

Liebert, R. M., & Morris, L. W. (1967). Cognitive and emotional components of test anxiety: A distinction and some initial data. *Psychological Reports, 20*, 975–978.

Morris, L. W., & Liebert, R. M. (1973). Effects of negative feedback, threat of shock, and level of trait anxiety on the arousal to two components of anxiety. *Journal of Consulting Psychology, 20*, 321–326.

Otto, J. (1982). Regulation und Fehlregulation im Verhalten VI. Anforderung und Kapazität beim Warten und beim Ausführen von Tätigkeiten [Behavioral regulation and dysregulation: VI. Demand and capacity during waiting and execution of activities]. *Psychologische Beiträge, 24*, 478–497.

Sarason, I. G. (1975). Anxiety and self-preoccupation. In I. G. Sarason & C. D. Spielberger (Eds.), *Stress and anxiety* (Vol. 2, pp. 27–44). Washington, DC: Hemisphere.

Schaefer, H., & Blohmke, M. (1977). *Herzkrank durch psychosozialen stress* [Heart diseases due to psychosocial stress]. Heidelberg, Federal Republic of Germany: Hüthig Verlag.

Schmidt, H. D. (1982). Die Situationshypertonie als Risikofaktor [Situational hypertension as a risk factor]. In D. Vaitl (Ed.), *Essentielle hypertonie* (pp. 77–111). Berlin, Federal Republic of Germany: Springer.

Schönpflug, W. (1983). *Anxiety, prospective orientation and preparation.* Invited paper presented at the conference "Stress and Anxiety," Warsaw, Poland.

Schulz, P., & Schönpflug, W. (1982). Regulatory activity during states of stress. In H. W. Krohne & L. Laux (Eds.), *Achievement, stress, and anxiety* (pp. 51–73). Washington, DC: Hemisphere.

Schwarzer, R. (1981). *Stress, Angst und Hilflosigkeit* [Stress, anxiety, and helplessness]. Stuttgart, Federal Republic of Germany: Kohlhammer.

Spielberger, C. D. (1972). Anxiety as an emotional state. In C. D. Spielberger (Ed.), *Anxiety: Current trends in theory and research* (Vol. 1, pp. 23–39). New York: Academic Press.

Spielberger, C. D. (1980). *Test anxiety inventory: Preliminary professional manual.* Palo Alto, CA: Consulting Psychologist Press.

Spielberger, C. D., Gonzalez, H. P., Taylor, C. J., Algaze, B., & Anton, W. D. (1978). Examination stress and test anxiety. In C. D. Spielberger & I. G. Sarason (Eds.), *Stress and anxiety* (Vol. 5, pp. 167–191). Washington, DC: Hemisphere.

Steptoe, A., Smulyan, H., & Gribbin, B. (1976). Pulse wave velocity and blood pressure change: Calibration and applications. *Psychophysiology, 13*(5), 488–493.

Weiner, B., & Potepan, P. A. (1970). Personality correlates and affective reactions towards exams of succeeding and failing college students. *Journal of Educational Psychology, 61,* 144–151.

Wieland, R., & Schönpflug, W. (1980). Regulation und Fehlregulation im Verhalten IV. Entspannung bei Angst und Lärmbelastung [Behavioral regulation and dysregulation: Relaxation, anxiety and noise]. *Psychologische Beiträge, 22,* 521–536.

Wine, J. (1971). Test anxiety and direction of attention. *Psychological Bulletin, 41,* 269–278.

Wine, J. (1982). Evaluation anxiety: A cognitive-attentional construct. In H. W. Krohne & L. Laux (Eds.), *Achievement, stress, and anxiety* (pp. 207–219). Washington, DC: Hemisphere.

Wortman, C. B., & Brehm, J. W. (1975). Responses to uncontrollable outcomes: An integration of reactance theory and the learned helplessness model. In L. Berkowitz (Ed.), *Advances in experimental social psychology* (Vol. 8, pp. 277–336). New York: Academic Press.

10

Self and Social Perceptions of Sport-Related Trait Anxiety

Dieter Hackfort
University of Heidelberg, Federal Republic of Germany

Empirical investigations have found significant discrepancies between self- and social perceptions of personality traits (see Shrauger & Schoeneman, 1979). For example, in an investigation of children's trait anxiety, Nickel and Schlüter (1970) found no correlations between self-ratings and teacher ratings of pupils' school anxiety. Children's and parents' ratings of children's achievement anxiety are also discrepant (see Helmke, 1979). Small but significant correlations were reported by Sarason, Davidson, Lighthall, Waite, and Ruebush (1960) in a validation study of the Test Anxiety Scale for Children. Similar results have been reported in studies that have used different anxiety inventories (e.g., Bottenberg & Moosbauer, 1975; Wieczerkowski, Nickel, Janowski, Fittkau, & Rauer, 1979).

Self- and social perceptions of anxiety are also discrepant in specific situations, such as sports competitions, when a general trait anxiety inventory is used, for example, the State–Trait Anxiety Inventory (STAI; Spielberger, Gorsuch, & Lushene, 1970). Hackfort and Schwenkmezger (1982) administered the STAI in a sport situation (gymnastic tasks) and found nonsignificant correlations between pupils' and teachers' ratings ranging between − .07 and .21. Moreover, the correlation coefficients in this study were not higher when anxiety was measured with Martens's (1977) Sport Competition Anxiety Test (SCAT), a sport-specific anxiety test. In an investigation of high school interscholastic girls' basketball teams, Martens and Simon (1976) found a correlation of .14 between SCAT scores and coaches' anxiety ratings. Similar findings were reported in a study of female volleyball players and their coaches (Martens, Rivkin, & Burton, 1980).

In analyzing these results, two points should be noted. First, in reviewing the methodology, it is important to note that the results are outcomes of correlational analyses with different kinds of data. Self-report data are based on perceptions related to the person's cognitions about his or her own affective state or disposition. Social perception data are based primarily on observations of behavior that are determined not only by emotions, but also by coping styles. This is especially true in social situations in which behavior is evaluated by others (e.g., parents, teachers, or coaches). There is also a tendency in social situations as well as in test situations to report behavior that is considered "socially desirable." Thus, the data of self-perception and social perception are at different distances from the anxiety construct. Sport-related anxiety as a subjective phenomenon can only be reported by the person who has the experience. Behavioral data require interpretation by an observer and are further removed from the construct.

Second, it is important to recognize that underlying the perception and valuations of other persons are so-called implicit theories of personality. These "naive theories" include subjective ideas about anxiety and anxiety-related dispositions that are integrated into a "naive concept of diagnosis" (see Hackfort, 1979, 1981). Such idiosyncratic concepts are not generally elaborated on or systematically tested and are often dominated by prejudices. Nevertheless, they regulate people's attention and actions in social situations.

Another explanation for the discrepancies between self- and social perceptions is suggested by attribution theory: According to the Jones-Nisbett (1971) hypothesis, there are two different kinds of causal attributions, depending on one's point of view: Actors see the causes of their behavior in terms of situational variables, whereas observers tend to regard personality traits as the sources of behavior. Favoring trait attributions over situational influences seems to be a fundamental attribution error (Ross, 1977).

One major cause of attribution errors may be that the actor and observer have different definitions of the situation because they have different relations with the given person–environment–task constellation (Hackfort, 1983). To act successfully requires attention to situational factors. In contrast, successful observation requires reduction of situational complexity, which can be facilitated by focusing on the interpretation of specific personal dispositions. The effectiveness of this strategy is supported by empirical results from Hackfort (1983), who found correlations of about .70 between teachers' ratings on five dimensions of sport-related anxiety in children (see also Hackfort, 1986). The correlation between these anxiety ratings and the children's grades was .50, indicating that a closer focus on more easily perceived and evaluated factors (e.g., sport performance) plays a critical role in social perceptions.

The accurate evaluation of sport-related anxiety by teachers is especially important in school settings because school experiences influence motivation to participate in leisure-time sports in later years. In the context of the findings and hypotheses I have outlined, a study was initiated to clarify the following questions:

1. Is there a relation between pupils' and teachers' anxiety ratings across different situations?
2. Is there a relation between self-rankings and social perception of sport-related anxiety in specific situations? (Are pupils with high or low self-report anxiety also judged by others as high or low in sport-related anxiety?)
3. Is there a relation between the definition of a situation and the discrepancy in self- and social perception? (Which ratings are more congruent, pupils' self-ratings with pupils' social ratings or pupils' self-ratings with teachers' social ratings of sport-related anxiety?)

METHOD

Subjects

The pupils were 60 male pupils aged 11–12 years and were selected from six school classes. The criterion for selection was that the pupil had been a member of the class for 2 years and had actively participated in the sports classes.

Instrument and Procedure

The instrument used to assess sport-related anxiety was a modification of the Sport Anxiety Diagnosis (SAD; Hackfort, 1983, 1986). Of the original set of 22 items, 5 items representing different sport-specific situations (trampoline, soccer, gymnastics, swimming, and high jump; Situations 1–5, respectively) were selected and administered with the special-answer category tables shown in Figures 1 and 2.

The pupils completed the SAD in two steps: First, they rated their own anxiety in each situation (self-perception, or SP). Second, they rated the anxiety of each of the other 9 pupils in the five situations (social perception by pupils, or SPP). In addition, the teachers rated the anxiety of each pupil in every situation (social perception by teachers, or SPT).

RESULTS AND DISCUSSION

The distributions of the ratings of SP, SPP, and SPT were evaluated by the Kolmogorov–Smirnov test. Significant deviations from the normal distribution were found in all cases (high anxiety was chosen less often than low anxiety). Therefore, the following statistical analyses were conducted using nonparametric procedures.

Anxiety levels measured for each of the three perspectives are reported in Table 1. The SP means were lower than the SPP means for all five situations, but higher than the SPT means. Especially interesting is the discrepancy between the SPP and SPT ratings. The pupils (SPP) gave significantly higher ratings of anxiety ($p <$ .001) than did the teachers (SPT) in all five situations, and tended to judge the anxiety level of their peers (SPP) as higher than their own (SP). These differences

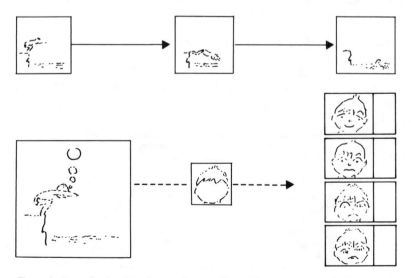

Figure 1   Example of an item from a sport-specific anxiety measurement: the Sport Anxiety Diagnosis (Hackfort, 1983).

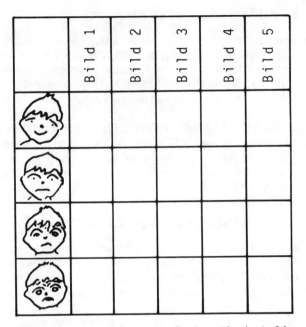

Figure 2   Answer-category table for five items (situations) of the
Sport Anxiety Diagnosis.

were significant ($p < .05$) in Situations 2 and 4. The significant differences between SP and SPT in Situations 3 ($p < .05$) and 5 ($p > .001$) showed that the
teachers did not recognize the pupils' anxiety level.

The teachers perceived less anxiety in their pupils than the pupils themselves
reported. Possible reasons for this are as follows:

1. The pupils know each other better than the teacher does because they have
more contact, communication, and interaction.

2. The pupils conceal their anxiety from the teacher but not from each other.

3. Pupils have a common perspective that is different from the teacher's point
of view.

Table 1   Mean Anxiety Level in Different Situations out
of Different Perception Perspectives

Situation	SP	SPP	SPT
Trampoline	1.83	1.92	1.41
Soccer	1.50	1.74	1.33
Gymnastics	1.96	2.07	1.63
Swimming	1.33	1.80	1.31
High jump	1.97	2.10	1.29
M	1.76	1.88	1.43

Note. SP = self-perception, SPP = social perception by
pupils, SPT = social perceptions by teachers.

4. Teachers do not like to recognize anxiety in their pupils, perhaps because they do not want to feel that their lessons are anxiety provoking.

5. It was also possible that the teachers' and pupils' standards for judging anxiety were different.

Another interesting finding was the hierarchy of the five situations for inducing anxiety from the three different perspectives. Only Situation 5 (high jump) was judged by the teachers as less anxiety inducing than the other situations, but this situation was judged as high anxiety inducing by the pupils. The pupils ranked Situation 3 (gymnastics) as second, Situation 1 (trampoline) third, and Situations 2 (soccer) and 4 (swimming) as fourth and fifth in terms of their anxiety-inducing potential.

Situation-Specific Analysis of Sport-Related Anxiety

To analyze situation-specific differences in self- and social perceptions of sport-related anxiety, Spearman correlation coefficients were computed between situations for each perception perspective. The correlations of self-perception between situations, reported in Table 2, ranged from .07 to .46. These small correlations demonstrate the specificity of the situations as separate sources of potential anxiety, as well as significant relations between anxiety perceptions for situations that have some structural similarity (Situations 1, 2, and 5 all include the task "jump up").

No significant correlation was found between self-perception of anxiety in soccer and gymnastics or trampoline (Situations 2 and 3 or 1). Moreover, the swimming and soccer situations did not seem to have a great potential for inducing anxiety (see Table 1).

Situational Specificity of Social Perceptions

To analyze the situational specificity of the social perceptions of anxiety, it is necessary to differentiate between the pupils' perspective and the teachers' perspective. Comparison of the correlations among the self-perceptions reported in Table 2 with those for the pupils' social perception in Table 3 shows that the social perceptions are much more highly correlated. The correlations among the pupils' social perceptions, which ranged from .73 to .87, were all highly significant.

Table 2 Spearman Correlation Coefficients between the Five Sport Situations for the Pupils' Self-Perception

Self-perception	1	2	3	4	5
Trampoline	—	.07	.31***	.21*	.46****
Soccer		—	.16	.24**	.21*
Gymnastics			—	.13	.33***
Swimming				—	.10
High jump					—

*$p \le$ .10.   **$p \le$ .05.   ***$p \le$ .01.   ****$p \le$ .001.

Table 3   Spearman Correlation Coefficients between the Five Sport
Situations for the Pupils' Social Perception

Social perception by pupils	1	2	3	4	5
Trampoline	—	.75	.77	.87	.77
Soccer		—	.76	.76	.75
Gymnastics			—	.81	.75
Swimming				—	.73
High jump					—

Note. $p \leq .001$ for all coefficients.

These results are consistent with the hypothesis that social perspective is oriented more toward personal dispositions than toward situation-specific factors.

The correlations among the teachers' social perceptions for the five situations are reported in Table 4. Although these correlations were not as high as those for the pupils' social perceptions (Table 3), they were higher than the correlations among the pupils' self-perceptions (Table 2), ranging from .46 to .74, and were all highly significant ($p < .001$), except for the correlation between the soccer and the swimming situations. The teachers' ratings seemed to be somewhat more situation specific than the pupils' social perceptions, but showed the same general tendency to reflect person-oriented judgments.

The low correlations between soccer and the other sport situations may reflect the difficulty of judging individual anxiety in a situation involving complex interactions among many persons. It is also possible that such game situations are less anxiety provoking. In summary, these results suggest that sport-related ratings of anxiety are determined by a person-centered orientation in social perception and by a more situational orientation in self-perception.

Cross-Situational Analysis of Sport-Related Anxiety

A cross-situational analysis of sport-related anxiety can be determined by computing a mean anxiety score over the five situations for each pupil, for each type of rating: SP, SPP, and SPT. The correlations between these mean anxiety scores (SPM, SPPM, SPTM) are shown in Table 5. The moderately high coefficients were all highly significant ($p < .001$). These findings are not surprising for the correlation between the two social perspectives (SPPM and SPTM), but they are

Table 4   Spearman Correlation Coefficients between the Five Sport
Situations for the Teachers' Social Perception

Social perceptions by teachers	1	2	3	4	5
Trampoline	—	.46**	.74**	.60**	.58**
Soccer		—	.49**	.29*	.49**
Gymnastics			—	.65**	.62**
Swimming				—	.65**
High jump					—

$*p \leq .10.$ $**p \leq .05.$

Table 5 Spearman Correlation Coefficients between
Mean Anxiety Scores for the Three Perspectives

Perspective	1	2	3
1. SPM	—	.47	.54
2. SPPM		—	.69
3. SPTM			—

Note. $p \leq .001$ for all coefficients. SPM = mean
self-perception, SPPM = mean social perception by
pupils, SPTM = mean social perception by teachers.

for the correlations between social perception and self-perception (SPM with
SPPM and SPM with SPTM).

These results support the hypothesis of a person-centered orientation in social
perception. The higher correlation of SPM with SPTM scores than with SPPM
scores suggests that teachers are more competent in rating anxious pupils than are
the pupils themselves (see also Alberti, 1971; Phillips, 1963). One main reason for
this might be the greater social distance between teachers and pupils than among
pupils.

Situation-Specific Conformity in Self- and Social Perceptions

The analysis of situation-specific conformity in self- and social perception in the
five specific sport situations was the final step in this investigation. Correlations
between the three perspectives for each situation, reported in Table 6, show that
the ratings were consistent in only one situation (swimming). The low correlations
of the SP ratings with the SPP and SPT ratings and the high correlations of the SPP
and SPT ratings are in line with the previously reported results.

SUMMARY AND CONCLUSIONS

In contrast to most previous investigations reviewed here, the results of this
study show significant positive correlations between self-perceptions and social
perceptions of anxiety. A major reason for these results may be the use of a

Table 6 Spearman Correlation Coefficients between the
Three Perspectives for the Five Sport Situations

Situation	SP–SPP	SP–SPT	SPP–SPT
Trampoline	.29*	.29*	.66***
Soccer	.04	.19	.44***
Gymnastics	.32**	.36**	.50***
Swimming	.45***	.45***	.69***
High jump	.11	.24*	.61***

Note. SP = self-perception, SPP = social perception by
pupils, SPT = social perception by teachers.
 *$p < .10$.   **$p < .05$.   ***$p < .01$.

situation-specific instrument, the SAD. Thus, the results underline the utility of situation-specific anxiety tests; these tests might also be helpful in school settings.

The most important findings of this study were the teachers' consistent underestimation of pupils' sport-related anxiety and the situational nonspecificity of the teachers' anxiety ratings. Two possible interpretations of these findings are considered. The first is that the recognition and evaluation of a negative disposition (anxiety is regarded as a negative disposition) requires more time than the evaluation of a neutral or positive disposition (Dorcus, 1926). Alternately, it is possible that teachers are not sensitive to emotional dispositions, such as trait anxiety.

This makes sense from a functional point of view because it is protective for the teachers: It protects them from doubts about their ability to organize a non-anxiety-provoking lesson from additional effort to provide special treatment for pupils with high anxiety, and so forth, and could be regarded as a social coping style similar to defensiveness (or repression).

Participation in sports is an important factor not only in leisure time activities, but also in the prevention and rehabilitation of illness (e.g., cardiac infarction). It is important to develop a positive motivation to engage in sport activities. However, anxiety hinders the development of such motivation in school. Therefore, teachers need to develop the ability and sensitivity to recognize sport-related anxiety in their pupils and to organize their lessons to help pupils overcome anxiety and encourage positive sport motivation.

REFERENCES

Alberti, J. M. (1971). Self-perception in school: Validation of an instrument and a study of the structure of children's self-perception-in-school and its relationship to school achievement, behavior and popularity. *Dissertation Abstracts International, 31,* 4535–4536A.

Bottenberg, E. H., & Moosbauer, W. (1975). Ängstlichkeit und Gedächtnisleistungen. Eine empirische Untersuchung an Kindern. [Trait anxiety and memory performance. An empirical investigation with children]. *Praxis der Kinderpsychologie und Kinderpsychiatrie, 24,* 1–6.

Dorcus, R. M. (1926). Some factors involved in judging personal characteristics. *Journal of Applied Psychology, 10,* 502–518.

Hackfort, D. (1979). *Grundlagen und Techniken der naiven Fremdbeeinflussung im Sport unter besonderer Berücksichtigung der Angstbeeinflussung* [Fundamentals and techniques of naive external control in sports: With special reference to anxiety control]. (Betrifft: Psychologie & Sport, Bd.5) Cologne, Federal Republic of Germany: Psychologisches Institut der Sporthochschule.

Hackfort, D. (1981). Naive Vorstellungen und Techniken der Angstkontrolle. [Naive concepts and techniques of anxiety control]. In W. Michaelis (Ed.), *Bericht über den 31. KongreB der Deutschen Gesellschaft für Psychologie in Zürich 1980, 2 Bde* (Vol. 1, pp. 681–686). Göttingen, Federal Republic of Germany: Hogrefe.

Hackfort, D. (1983). *Theorie und Diagnostik sportbezogener Ängstlichkeit—Ein situationsalytischer Ansatz.* [Theory and diagnosis of sport-related anxiety—A situational analytical concept]. Unveröff. Diss. DSHS Köln.

Hackfort, D. (1986). Theoretical conception and assessment of sport-related anxiety. In C. D. Spielberger & R. Diaz-Guerrero (Eds.), *Cross-cultural anxiety* (Vol. 3, pp. 79–88). New York: Hemisphere/McGraw-Hill.

Hackfort, D., & Schwenkmezger, P. (1982). Psychologische Aspekte zur Angst im Sportunterricht. [Psychological aspects of anxiety in physical education classes]. *Sportunterricht, 11,* 409–419.

Helmke, A. (1979). Elterliche Diagnosefähigkeit: Zur Frage des Zusammenhangs zwischen kindlicher Selbstwahrnehmung von Leistungsangst und Beurteilungen durch die Eltern. [Parents' diagnostic ability: Correlational aspects to the self perception of the child's achievement anxiety and the judgment of the parents]. In H. W. Krohne & R. Schaffner (Eds.), *Entwicklungsbedingungen von Angst und Anstabwehr* (pp. 19–25). Psychologische Forschungsberichte aus dem Fachbereich 3 der Universität Osnabrück, Nr. 14.

Jones, E. E., & Nisbett, R. E. (1971). *The actor and the observer: Divergent perceptions of the causes of behavior.* Morristown, NJ: General Learning Press.

Martens, R. (1977). *Sport competition anxiety test.* Champaign, IL: Human Kinetics Publishers.

Martens, R., & Simon, J. A. (1976). Comparison of three predictors of state anxiety in competitive situations. *Research Quarterly, 47,* 381–387.

Martens, R., Rivkin, F., & Burton, D. (1980). Who predicts anxiety better: Coaches or athletes? In C. H. Nadeu, W. R. Halliwell, K. M. Newell, & G. C. Roberts (Eds.), *Psychology of motor behavior and sport—1979* (pp. 84–90). Champaign, IL: Human Kinetics Publishers.

Nickel, H., & Schlüter, P. (1970). Angstwerte bei Hauptschülern und ihr Zusammenhang mit Leistungst-sowie Verhaltensmerkmalen, Lehrerurteil und Unterrichtsstil. [Anxiety scores of pupils and correlations with performance and behavior, teachers' judgment, and style of teaching]. *Zeitschrift für Entwicklungspsychologie und Pädagogische Psychologie, 2,* 125–136.

Phillips, B. N. (1963). Age changes in accuracy of self-perception. *Child Development, 64,* 1041–1046.

Ross, L. (1977). The intuitive psychologist and his shortcomings: Distortions in the attribution process. In L. Berkowitz (Ed.), *Advances in experimental social psychology, Vol. 10* (pp. 173–220). New York: Academic Press.

Sarason, S. B., Davidson, K. S., Lighthall, F. F., Waite, R. R., & Ruebush, B. K. (1960). *Anxiety in elementary school children.* New York: Wiley.

Shrauger, J. S., & Schoeneman, T. J. (1979). Symbolic interactionist view of self-concept: Through the looking glass darkly. *Psychological Bulletin, 86,* 549–573.

Spielberger, C. D., Gorsuch, R. L., & Lushene, R. E. (1970). *Manual for the State–Trait Anxiety Inventory (STAI).* Palo Alto, CA: Consulting Psychologists Press.

Wieczerkowski, W., Nickel, H., Janoswki, A., Fittkau, R., & Rauer, W. (1979). *Angstfragebogen für Schüler (AFS).* [Anxiety inventory for pupils]. Göttingen, Federal Republic of Germany: Hogrefe.

11

Application of Stress Inoculation Training for the Treatment of Test Anxiety

Mildred Vera and José J. Bauermeister
University of Puerto Rico

The debilitating effects of test anxiety have been extensively documented (Sarason, 1980). Students with high scores on measures of test anxiety demonstrate a poorer performance on cognitive laboratory tasks and on intelligence and achievement tests, as well as administered exams in the classroom (e.g., Deffenbacher, 1980; Dusek, 1980; Wine, 1980). Evaluation anxiety is a pervasive phenomenon. It is estimated that approximately 10% of the male and 12% of the female high school student population in Puerto Rico experience high levels of test anxiety and identify this emotional reaction as a significant problem in their lives (Bauermeister, 1989). In spite of its importance, there are no published studies on the treatment of test anxiety for Puerto Rican students or students from other Spanish-speaking countries. This chapter responds to this need and examines the effectiveness of stress inoculation training (Meichenbaum, 1975) for the treatment of test anxiety in high school students.

Both theory and research suggest that the concept of test anxiety refers to individual differences in the predisposition to respond with emotional reactions and self-centered worry cognitions when confronted with evaluative situations (Alpert & Haber, 1960; Mandler & Sarason, 1952, 1953; Morris & Liebert, 1970; Sarason, 1960, 1975, 1980; Spielberger, Anton, & Bedell, 1976; Spielberger, González, Taylor, Algaze, & Anton, 1978; Suinn, 1969; Wine, 1971). Emotional reactions are characterized by feelings of tension, apprehension, nervousness, and the activation of the autonomic nervous system. Worry cognitions are related to self-critical and self-derogatory task-irrelevant thoughts (Morris & Liebert, 1970; Sarason, 1960, 1972, 1975; Spielberger et al., 1976; Wine, 1971). Most researchers agree that these worry cognitions significantly interfere with performance on tests (Morris & Liebert, 1970; Sarason, 1960, 1972, 1975; Wine, 1971, 1980). From a therapeutic viewpoint, the findings of these researchers, and the theories that have been developed, point to the importance of including procedures that can modify the student's tendency to engage in self-centered worry cognitions and emotional reactions.

This research was supported in part by the University of Puerto Rico Institutional Research Fund to José J. Bauermeister.

Part of this research was submitted by Mildred Vera in partial fulfillment for a master's degree at the University of Puerto Rico, Río Piedras Campus.

We gratefully acknowledge the assistance provided by Margarita Alegría and María Miranda.

It has been reported that test anxiety is negatively correlated with study habits in students from the United States (Allen, Lerner, & Hinrichsen, 1972; Wittmaier, 1972) and from Puerto Rico (Bauermeister, Collazo, & Spielberger, 1983; Bauermeister, Huergo, García, & Otero, 1988). Thus, it is necessary to include training in study habits in the treatment of test anxiety.

The stress inoculation training procedure (Meichenbaum, 1975; Meichenbaum & Cameron, 1983) facilitates the inclusion of multimodal therapeutic techniques that can help students to modify the predisposition to engage in worry cognitions and emotionality reactions and to develop coping skills, such as relaxation techniques and study habits. This treatment method can also enhance the students' motivation to use the skills learned during therapy to cope actively with the inherent stress in the testing situation. These aspects have not been considered adequately in previous research on the treatment of test anxiety (Spielberger, González, & Fletcher, 1979).

The goals of stress inoculation training are that the participants (a) understand the nature of the events that contribute to their emotional reactions, (b) learn appropriate behaviors to cope with the source of stress, and (c) practice and apply these newly learned skills in stressful situations (Meichenbaum, 1975; Meichenbaum & Cameron, 1983, Meichenbaum, Turk, & Burstein, 1975; Novaco, 1979). Operationally, the treatment consists of three phases. The first is of an educational nature. Through group discussions, the participants are provided with a conceptual framework that helps them to visualize and understand their emotional reactions. In this conceptualization, the emphasis is on the fact that the emotional reactions associated with a stressful situation are influenced by the way the situation is perceived and the course of action that is taken in relation to it, not by the situation per se. In the second phase, the participants acquire and rehearse various skills to cope with the stressful situation. The most important skill is cognitive restructuring: The participants learn to identify and analyze the maladaptive, irrational thoughts that evoke anxiety when one is faced with stressful situations, and to replace these thoughts with incompatible coping self-statements. In the third phase, the participants apply their newly learned coping skills while exposed to stressful situations (Meichenbaum, 1975; Meichenbaum & Cameron, 1983; Meichenbaum et al., 1975; Novaco, 1979).

Stress inoculation training has been shown to be effective for the treatment of medical problems, such as enhancing pain control (Turk, 1976; Wells, Howard, Nowlin, & Vargas, 1986); anger reactions (Feindler & Fremouw, 1983; Novaco, 1977); and terrorist and rape victims (Ayalon, 1983; Veronen & Kilpatrick, 1983). Hussian and Lawrence (1978) demonstrated that this procedure can be effective for the treatment of test anxiety in U.S. college students. However, this study has been criticized for its lack of emphasis on adequately developing the third phase of treatment application (Novaco, 1979).

In the treatment designed for the present study, students are helped to understand the factors that contribute to their test anxiety reactions. The students are also provided with the opportunity to learn, practice, and use skills to cope with the stress produced by the test situation. Some of these skills were the identification, analysis, and modification of their task-irrelevant worry thoughts; muscular relaxation; and study habits, work methods, and strategies to answer tests, among others. These procedures are described in the next section.

METHOD

Participants

The participants were 32 (16 male and 16 female) high school students, of whom 16 were assigned to the treatment groups and 16 were assigned to the control groups. The participants were 9th-, 10th-, and 11th-grade students who were enrolled in a private school in San Juan, Puerto Rico. Their ages ranged from 13 to 16 years.

Participant Selection

The students were selected on the basis of their scores on the *Inventario de Auto-Evaluación Sobre Exámenes* (IDASE), which was administered to all high school students. The IDASE has been developed to assess individual differences in the predisposition to experience emotional reactions and worry cognitions in test situations (Bauermeister et al., 1983, 1988). The IDASE consists of a 20-item questionnaire that asks the respondent to describe how he or she generally feels in test situations. It includes two subscales to assess emotionality and worry reactions. The IDASE is the Spanish version of the Test Anxiety Inventory (Spielberger et al., 1978).

The students who were selected met the following criteria: (a) IDASE total scores that corresponded to a percentile rank of 75 or more, according to the norms obtained for Puerto Rican high school students (Bauermeister et al., 1988); (b) a confirmation, on the basis of the students' response to a questionnaire, that test anxiety was a serious problem for them; and (c) an expressed interest in participating in a treatment program for test anxiety. Of a total of 207 students who were assessed, 46 met this criteria.

Pretreatment Evaluation

Instruments

The participants were administered the *Inventario de Preocupación y Emocionalidad Ante la Situación de Examen* (IPEASE), the Spanish version of the Study Habits Scale of the Survey of Study Habits and Attitudes (*Encuesta de Hábitos y Actitudes hacia el Estudio–Forma P*; Brown & Holtzman, 1975), and the A-Trait scale of the Inventario de Ansiedad, Rasgo y Estado (IDARE; Spielberger, González, Martínez, Natalicio, & Natalicio, 1971).

The IPEASE is an inventory developed to assess the frequency with which students report anxiety and worry reactions when faced with tests (Bauermeister, 1986). This inventory includes an Emotionality and Worry Scale. As with the IDASE, the IPEASE provides a measure of trait anxiety specific to the test situation.

The Study Habits (SH) Scale combines the scores on the Delay Avoidance (DA) and Work Methods (WM) scales to provide a measure of academic behavior. The DA Scale measures the promptness in completing academic assignments, lack of procrastination, and freedom from delay and distraction. The WM Scale measures the use of effective study procedures, efficiency in doing academic assignments, and study skills (Brown & Holtzman, 1975).

The A-Trait Scale of the IDARE measures the predisposition to experience anxiety reactions. Students with a high level of A-Trait demonstrate a greater predisposition to perceive a wide range of stimulus as threatening and to respond to such threats with greater elevations in state anxiety, as compared with students with a low level of A-Trait (Spielberger et al., 1971).

As a measure of academic achievement, the grade-point averages (GPAs) of the participants were obtained for the following courses: Spanish, English, mathematics, and history. The GPAs were calculated for the trimester that ended before the initiation of the treatment program.

Group Formation

Two treatment groups of 9 students each were organized.[1] These groups were labeled *treatment male* (TM) and *treatment female* (TF). The students in these groups were randomly selected from among those who, in addition to meeting the criteria previously identified, shared a free time period during the school day to participate in the treatment program. Two control groups of 8 students each were formed: control male (CM) and control female (CF). The control group participants were also randomly selected from among the students who met the selection criteria; however, these students did not have a common free period in which to meet and to participate in the treatment program.

Treatment

The students assigned to the TM and TF groups were subdivided into two groups. Each subgroup consisted of four men and women. These subgroups participated twice a week in a treatment program that consisted of 12 sessions, each 50 min long. The CM and CF groups were evaluated before and after treatment, but did not receive any type of therapeutic intervention.

The therapist had a master's degree in counseling psychology and six years of experience as a teacher and high school counselor. She was also a second-year clinical psychology graduate student and had approved courses, laboratory experiences, and supervised practice in group therapy and behavior modification. In two of the sessions, another female therapist, who was also a graduate student with similar training, modeled strategies of how to cope with test situations. A university professor, with experiences in the area of assessment and treatment of test anxiety, supervised the therapists through tape recordings of the sessions and periodic meetings.

The stress inoculation treatment was divided into three phases. These are briefly described.

First Phase: Cognitive Preparation

This phase consisted of two sessions. The goal was to develop in the participants an understanding of the conceptual framework of the test anxiety reactions. In the first session, the therapist guided the group discussion around the kind of thoughts and feelings that are experienced while taking tests. Through this discus-

---

[1]One of the students did not complete the treatment and another was randomly eliminated in order to have an equal number of participants per group ($n = 8$).

sion, the experiences described by the students were used so that the participants could understand (a) how their anxiety reactions were associated with the way they perceived the test situation; (b) how irrational, maladaptive thoughts evoke anxiety; and (c) how self-centered worry thoughts interfere with performance on tests. In the second session, the students discussed the antecedents, frequency, duration, and content of their maladaptive thoughts in test-taking situations. The experiences discussed were related to worry cognitions concerning (a) performance on tests ("I'm going to forget everything"), (b) psychophysiological reactions that accompany anxiety (increased heart rate), (c) the possible consequences of failing the test (punishment, disapproval), and (d) inadequacy or self-criticism ("I'm stupid"). The discussion of these experiences was further aimed at helping the participants become aware of their worry cognitions and the effect these cognitions had on their behavior in test situations.

Second Phase: Skills Rehearsal

This phase consisted of eight sessions. The goal was to help the participants become aware of the type of thoughts that evoke anxiety in evaluative situations and to replace these thoughts with incompatible self-statements. Other skills developed in this phase were relaxation and study habits.

In the third and fourth sessions, the therapist directed the group discussion around the content of the egocentric worry reactions that the participants had identified while in evaluative situations. Through the use of participant modeling and role playing, different examples of incompatible self-statements that could be used to contend with worry cognitions were demonstrated. The participants were taught muscular relaxation, deep-breathing exercises, and self-instructions to cope with anxiety reactions in evaluative situations. They were also asked to practice the muscle relaxation exercises at least once a day. In the fifth session, the discussion on maladaptive thoughts and their impact on evaluative situations was continued. Relaxation exercises were practiced. In this session, the need to improve study habits and skills and the importance of organizing available study time efficiently were emphasized. The students were taught how to design a program of daily activities that included a study period. The participants designed their own program of activities.

During the 6th–10th sessions, the relaxation exercises were practiced. The participants were also taught an accelerated method of muscle and self-instructed relaxation. Group discussion continued on becoming aware of maladaptive, self-centered, worry responses and the substitution of the latter with incompatible coping self-statements. The following topics were covered: strategies for memory improvement, classroom note-taking, and ways to prepare chapter summaries. Students practiced these study skills and discussed strategies for answering different types of tests. In the last two sessions, a coping modeling procedure (Bauermeister & Ouslán, 1974) was used to demonstrate how to manage anxiety and worry reactions. In these sessions, another therapist performed as a model, verbalizing feelings of anxiety and worry as she was ready to take a test. This model identified the physiological reactions that accompanied her feelings of anxiety. In addition, she verbalized maladaptive, task-irrelevant worry self-statements. The model then proceeded to demonstrate skills and strategies to cope with test anxiety.

Examples of these strategies are brief muscular relaxation, deep breathing, coping self-statements, and self-reinforcement.

Third Phase: Treatment Application

In this last phase, which included the last two sessions, the participants were offered the opportunity to practice the skills that had previously been learned in a simulated test situation. In addition, students were encouraged to continue practicing these skills while studying and taking tests. For the simulated situation, a mathematics teacher participated in one of the sessions and assigned different algebra exercises. This particular teacher was perceived by the students as being highly demanding and strict. Subsequently, she approached each student and corrected the work. The teacher proceeded to discuss the exercises and then administered a test. Although the participants knew that the score on this test was not going to be included in their course grade, pressure was exerted by shortening the time available to complete the test and through a variety of comments. On completing the test, the participants shared their experiences and the strategies they used to cope with their anxiety reactions.

Posttreatment Evaluation

Two research assistants readministered the instruments that were used in the pretreatment evaluation phase. This evaluation was performed a week after the treatment was terminated.

Follow-Up Evaluation

The follow-up evaluation was performed 2 months after the treatment was completed. The IPEASE was administered by the teachers immediately before a final exam. It was not possible to administer the other instruments because of time limitations.

RESULTS

The mean scores obtained by the treatment and control groups in the pretreatment and posttreatment evaluation phase are presented in Table 1. In general, the TM and TF groups obtained lower posttreatment mean scores on the test anxiety and A-Trait measures, relative to (a) their respective pretreatment scores and (b) the posttreatment scores of the CM and CF groups. On the other hand, the TM and TF groups obtained higher posttreatment mean scores on the study habits measures, as can be seen in Table 1.

A factorial analysis of covariance (ANCOVA; Kerlinger & Pedhazur, 1973) was performed for each of the posttreatment scores. The following were used as covariables: (a) scores obtained by the groups in the pretreatment evaluation phase, (b) school grade (9th, 10th, or 11th), and (c) a combination of the pretreatment scores and school grade. The covariables analyzed were not statistically significant ($p > .05$) for the following measures: the IDASE and IPEASE Emotionality scales; and the WM Scale of the Study Habits Scale. For these variables, a factorial analysis of variance (ANOVA) was performed (Glass & Stanley, 1970). In the

Table 1 Scores Obtained by the Treatment Male (TM), Treatment Female (TF), Control Male (CM), and Control Female (CF) Groups in the Pretreatment and Posttreatment Evaluation

	Group							
	TM		TF		CM		CF	
Measure	Pretreatment	Posttreatment	Pretreatment	Posttreatment	Pretreatment	Posttreatment	Pretreatment	Posttreatment
IDASE	53.27	39.63	64.62	36.38	54.00	51.50	57.50	58.75
Emotionality (IDASE)	16.62	12.13	19.87	10.25	16.75	16.25	17.75	17.63
Worry (IDASE)[a]	15.62	11.32	17.37	9.58	15.25	13.65	15.62	17.06
Emotionality (IPEASE)	35.50	26.88	39.62	27.75	33.25	33.00	33.62	36.00
Worry (IPEASE)[a]	90.87	73.63	89.75	59.13	79.62	74.13	83.62	89.50
Study habits	30.37	45.16	43.00	52.33	36.25	41.61	47.50	40.89
Delay avoidance[a]	12.12	27.95	19.37	32.58	17.25	10.33	22.62	25.76
Work methods	18.25	21.25	23.62	29.13	19.00	20.50	24.87	25.75
A-Trait[a]	50.00	43.63	52.62	44.13	48.62	44.88	45.75	51.88

Note. IDASE = *Inventario de Auto-Evaluacion Sobre Exámenes,* IPEASE = *Inventario de Preocupacion y Emocionalidad Ante la Situacion de Examen.*
[a]For these variables, the mean scores have been corrected, taking into consideration the significant effects of the covariables used in the analysis.

ANCOVAs and ANOVAs performed, treatment and sex of the participants were treated as independent variables.

Test Anxiety Measures

Table 2 presents a summary of the findings of the ANOVA for the IDASE scores. Statistically significant treatment effects were obtained. The IDASE posttreatment scores of the TM and TF groups were significantly lower than those of the CM and CF groups, as can be observed in Tables 1 and 2. Similar findings were obtained for the IDASE Emotionality Scale, $F(1, 28) = 15.18, p < .001$. An examination of Table 1 further indicates that the TM and TF groups also obtained lower mean scores on the Emotionality Scale of the IPEASE. These differences were significant, $F(1, 28) = 6.14, p < .05$. No significant Sex × Treatment effects were found in these analyses of the two emotionality scales.

The ANCOVA for the IDASE Worry Scale demonstrated significant treatment effects, $F(1, 27) = 16.21, p < .001$, and Sex × Treatment effects $F(1, 27) = 4.77, p < .05$. Analysis of the data presented in Table 1 suggests that the stress inoculation training was more effective for the TF group than for the TM group. This was confirmed by post hoc analyses with the Tukey test, which indicated that the TF group scores were significantly lower than the CF group scores ($q = 7.48$, $p < .01$). No other group differences were found. Similar findings were obtained in the ANCOVA for the IPEASE Worry Scale. Treatment, $F(1, 27) = 19.20, p < .001$, and Sex × Treatment effects, $F(1, 27) = 6.71, p < .05$, were significant. The TF group scores were significantly lower than the CF group scores ($q = 34.23, p < .01$).

Study Habits Measure

The ANCOVA for the SH Scale yielded significant treatment effects. The SH Scale scores for the TM and TF groups were significantly higher than the scores for the CM and CF groups, as is evident from Tables 1 and 2. Significant treatment effects were also obtained for scores on the DA scale, $F(1, 27) = 5.38, p < .05$. The ANOVA for the scores on the WM Scale demonstrated significant effects for sex

Table 2 Summary of the Analyses of Variance and Covariance for the Scores on the Inventario de Autoevaluación Sobre Exámenes (IDASE), Study Habits, and A-Trait.

Source of variation	df	IDASE		Study habits		A-Trait	
		MS	F	MS	F	MS	F
Main effect	2	1189.1	7.81*	266.1	2.75	258.4	6.02**
Sex	1	32.0	0.21	71.2	0.74	117.5	2.73
Treatment	1	2346.1	15.41*	436.7	4.51*	399.9	9.32**
Sex × Treatment	1	220.5	1.45	124.6	1.29	210.3	4.90*
Residual	28	152.3		96.9		42.9	

Note. An analysis of variance was done for the IDASE scores, and the *df* for the residual error term was 27.

*$p < .05$.   ** $p < .01$.

only, $F(1, 28) = 4.59$, $p < .05$. The female participants obtained higher scores than the male participants, as can be seen in Table 1.

Trait Anxiety Measure

As it is evident from Table 2, the ANCOVA yielded significant treatment and Sex × Treatment effects. The Tukey test indicated significant differences between the A-Trait scores of the TF and CF groups ($q = 11.70$, $p < .01$). These data are indicative that the treatment effects were specific to the female participants who received the stress inoculation training.

Academic Achievement Measures

The overall GPA for the fourth trimester was used as the posttreatment measure. The ANCOVA did not yield any treatment or interaction effects for this posttreatment measure of academic achievement ($p > .05$). A significant Sex × Treatment interaction effect was obtained for the mathematics GPA, $F(1, 27) = 5.57$, $p < .05$. The Tukey test indicated that the TM group had a higher trimester grade than the TF group ($q = 8.41$, $p < .05$). No other group differences were found. A significant Sex × Treatment interaction was also found for the GPA in the history course, $F(1, 27) = 4.77$, $p < .05$. The Tukey test indicated significant differences between the TM and CM groups only ($q = 8.74$, $p < .05$). These findings indicate that the stress inoculation training was effective in improving the GPA of the TM group in the mathematics and history courses, respectively. Table 3 presents the GPA obtained by the participants in these two courses.

No significant findings were obtained for the ANCOVA of the posttreatment grades in the English and Spanish courses ($p > .05$).

Follow-Up Measures

The IPEASE Emotionality and Worry Scales were administered 2 months after treatment completion, immediately before a final exam. Table 4 presents the means obtained. For the Emotionality Scale, the ANOVA demonstrated significant treatment effects, $F(1, 23) = 9.95$, $p < .01$. The means of the TM and TF groups were lower than the means of the CM and CF groups.

For the Worry Scale, the ANCOVA demonstrated a significant Sex × Treatment interaction, $F(1, 23) = 15.87$, $p < .001$. The Tukey test indicated the presence of significant differences ($p < .05$) between the TM and CM groups ($q = 16.22$), TF and CF groups ($q = 52.90$), and TM and TF groups ($q = 17.23$). These analyses indicate that the stress inoculation training was effective in reducing worry reactions for both the male and female participants, but had a greater effect on the latter.

DISCUSSION

This study examined the effectiveness of the stress inoculation training procedure (Meichenbaum, 1975; Meichenbaum & Cameron, 1983; Meichenbaum et al., 1975) for the treatment of test anxiety in Puerto Rican high school students. Pre-

Table 3 Mean Scores for the History and Mathematics
Courses Obtained in the Posttreatment
Evaluation

	Course	
Group	Mathematics	History
Treatment male	80.97	80.74
Treatment female	72.56	82.69
Control male	73.90	72.27
Control female	73.96	78.86

vious research on the treatment of test anxiety in the United States points to the importance of including therapeutic procedures that can modify students' tendency to experience self-centered worry and emotional responses in evaluative situations (Morris & Liebert, 1970; Sarason, 1960, 1975, 1980; Spielberger et al., 1976; Spielberger et al. 1979; Wine, 1971, 1980). Other studies have underscored the importance of including training on study habits and skills in the treatment of test anxiety (Allen et al., 1972; Lent & Rusell, 1978; Mitchell & Ng, 1972; Wittmaier, 1972). Finally, the importance of motivating students to apply the skills learned during treatment in test situations has been emphasized (Spielberger et al., 1979). Stress inoculation training was selected as a treatment procedure because it provides the flexibility for the design of a multimodal treatment that includes the issues previously pointed out.

In this treatment program, group discussions were guided by the therapist so as to help the students become aware that their difficulties in test situations were related to task-irrelevant, self-centered worry cognitions. The group discussions were further aimed at analyzing these worry cognitions and developing strategies for replacing the latter with incompatible coping self-statements that could help the students direct their attention to the test tasks. These procedures were also modeled by the therapist and practiced by the participants. Relaxation, study, and test-taking skills were also taught. These skills were practiced in both simulated and real test situations.

The results of the present investigation demonstrate that stress inoculation training is an effective method for the treatment of test anxiety in Puerto Rican students. The students assigned to the treatment condition obtained significantly

Table 4 Mean Scores for the Emotionality and Worry Scales of the *Inventario de Preocupación y Emocionalidad Ante la Situación de Exámen* Obtained in the Follow-Up Evaluation Completed 2 Months after Treatment Termination

	Group			
Measure	Treatment male	Treatment female	Control male	Control female
Emotionality Scale	24.86	24.86	34.71	38.86
Worry Scale[a]	59.64	44.76	74.33	96.76

[a]For this variable, the means have been adjusted, taking into consideration the significant effects of the covariables.

lower IDASE scores on treatment completion than did the control groups. These findings suggest that stress inoculation training decreased the predisposition of the participants to perceive the test situation as threatening and to react with increases in state anxiety and self-centered, task-irrelevant thoughts. The scores of the participants assigned to the treatment condition on the IDASE and IPEASE Emotionality scales, respectively, were also significantly lower. Both instruments assess the students' predisposition to experience emotional reactions in test situations, that is, feelings of restlessness, anxiety, tension, and panic and increases in heart rate (Bauermeister, 1986; Bauermeister et al. 1988). However, a significant Treatment × Sex interaction effect was obtained for the IDASE and IPEASE Worry scales, respectively. These findings suggest that for this measure, the stress inoculation training was effective for the female students only. The IDASE Worry Scale provides a measure of students' predisposition to anticipate failure and its consequences, to distract themselves with task-irrelevant cognitions, and to engage in self-devaluative thoughts (Bauermeister et al., 1988). The IPEASE Worry Scale measures similar reactions (Bauermeister, 1986).

Additional evidence on the effectiveness of the stress inoculation training is obtained from the emotionality and worry measures of the IPEASE, administered 2 months after treatment completion, immediately after a final exam. In this evaluation, the male treatment group obtained significantly lower scores than did the male control group. These findings are indicative that by the time the follow-up measure were taken, the treatment was also effective in reducing the predisposition to worry in the male participants. The treatment effects, however, were of a greater magnitude for the female participants.

A significant Treatment × Sex interaction effect was also obtained for the IDARE A-Trait Scale. Stress inoculation training was found to be effective in reducing the A-Trait scores of the female participants only. This scale measures the predisposition to perceive a wide variety of situations as threatening and to respond to such threats with increases in state anxiety (Spielberger et al., 1971). The reduction in A-Trait is consistent with the modification of worry responses for the female participants assigned to the treatment condition.

A possible explanation for these differential treatment effects is that the discussion and modeling of the skills necessary to cope with task-irrelevant worry cognitions caught the attention of the participants who were the same sex as the therapists more (i.e., the female students). It has been reported that subjects pay more attention to those models they perceived as being more similar to them or who are of the same sex (Bandura, 1969; Rohrbaugh, 1979), and that a model's efficiency in transmitting behaviors through imitation increases when the observers perceive themselves as similar to the model (Flanders, 1968). Thus, it is possible that the female participants perceived the intervention and modeling of the therapists as more pertinent to their experience, and that this perception facilitated the treatment effects. This hypothesis is supported by the results of the evaluation questionnaire administered at the end of treatment. It was found that 63% of the female participants indicated that the topics relating to the way thoughts interfere with the performance in tests had been discussed and practiced very effectively. The remaining 37% of the female participants evaluated this discussion and practice as effective. In contrast, 25% of the men evaluated the discussion of these topics as very effective, 50% evaluated it as effective, and 25% evaluated it as average.

Independent of the reasons, the interactions obtained for the worry and A-Trait measures are of particular theoretical and clinical interest. These interactions suggest that for Puerto Rican students, the effectiveness of stress inoculation training can vary depending on the sex of the participants and of the therapist. Further research is needed to clarify this important issue.

The scores obtained by the students assigned to the treatment condition on the SH Scale (Brown & Holtzman, 1975) were significantly higher than the scores of the control groups. Further analysis of this measure indicated that the treatment groups obtained significantly higher scores on the DA Scale than the control groups. These findings suggest that the stress inoculation training was effective in increasing the students' promptness in completing academic assignments free from wasteful delay and distractions (Brown & Holtzman, 1975). In contrast, no significant differences were found for scores on the WM Scale between the treatment and control groups. The latter assesses effective study procedures, efficiency in doing academic assignments, and how-to-study skills (Brown & Holtzman, 1975). It is possible that the discussion of these topics was covered too late in the treatment program and that insufficient time was given for the participants to improve their study methods.

No statistically significant differences were found for the overall GPA of the treatment and control groups. Significant Treatment × Sex interaction effects were found for the GPAs obtained in the mathematics and history courses, respectively. Only the male students significantly improved their grades on these subject matters. These findings, in addition to the Treatment × Sex interaction found for the worry and A-Trait measures, point to the complexity of the relation between test anxiety reduction and improvement in academic achievement.

In future research, it will be necessary to expand the activities designed to develop study methods. It is also necessary to revise the point in time at which the measurements of these skills, and the GPA of the participants, are obtained. Denny and Rupert (1977), for example, reported that no significant findings were obtained in students' GPAs during the semester in which treatment was applied. However, in subsequent semesters, significant differences were obtained between the experimental and control groups.

It has been reported that the predisposition to experience anxiety in test situations affects a considerable number of Puerto Rican students (Bauermeister, 1989). Although this predisposition is described as a serious problem, the students seek their friends more than school personnel for counseling. The stress inoculation procedures used in this study can serve as a model for the development of a treatment program for this population, as it effectively makes use of peer assistance. This treatment can be applied by school personnel such as counselors, psychologists, social workers, and properly trained teachers. In future application of this treatment, it will be necessary to expand the activities addressed to development of study methods, and to revise the cognitive activities to be discussed and modeled, taking into consideration the sex of the therapist and of the participants.

REFERENCES

Allen, G. J., Lerner, W. M., & Hinrichsen, J. J. (1972). Study behaviors and their relationships to test anxiety and academic performance. *Psychological Reports, 30,* 407–410.

Alpert, R., & Haber, R. M. (1960). Anxiety in academic achievement situation. *Journal of Abnormal and Social Behavior, 61,* 207–215.

Ayalon. O. (1983). Coping with terrorism. The Israeli case. In D. Meichenbaum & M. E. Jaremko (Eds.), *Stress reduction and prevention* (pp. 293–339). New York: Plenum Press.

Bandura, A. (1969). *Principles of behavior modification.* New York: Holt, Rinehart & Winston.

Bauermeister, J. J. (1986). *Confiabilidad y validez del Inventario de Preocupación y Emocionalidad ante la Situación de Examen (IPEASE)* [Reliability and validity of the Worry and Emotionality Test Anxiety Inventory]. Unpublished manuscript.

Bauermeister, J. J. (1989). Estrés de evaluación y reacciones de ansiedad ante la situación de examen [Evaluation stress and anxiety reactions to test situations]. *Avances en Psicología Clínica Latinoamericana 7,* 69–88.

Bauermeister, J. J., Collazo, J. A., & Spielberger, C. D. (1983). The construction and validation of the Spanish form of the Test Anxiety Inventory: Inventario de Auto-Evaluación sobre Exámenes (IDASE). In C. D. Spielberger & R. Díaz-Guerrero (Eds.), *Cross-cultural anxiety* (Vol. 2, pp. 67–85). New York: Hemisphere/McGraw-Hill.

Bauermeister, J. J., Huergo, M., García, C. I., & Otero, R. (1988). El Inventario de Auto-Evaluación Sobre Exámenes (IDASE) y su aplicabilidad a estudiantes de escuela secundaria [Applicability of the IDASE to secondary school students]. *Hispanic Journal of Behavioral Sciences, 10,* 21–37.

Bauermeister, J. J., & Ouslán, A. (1974). *Comparación de los efectos de modelado en niños* [Comparison of modeling effects on children]. Presentation before the InterAmerican Congress of Psychology, Bogotá, Colombia.

Brown, W. F., & Holtzman, W. H. (1975). *Encuesta de Hábitos y Actitudes Hacia el Estudio* [Survey of Study Habits and Attitudes]. Ciudad, México: Editorial Trillas.

Deffenbacher, J. L. (1980). Worry and emotionality in test anxiety. In I. G. Sarason (Ed.), *Test anxiety: Theory, research, and application* (pp. 111–128). Hillsdale, NJ: Erlbaum.

Denny, D. R., & Rupert, P. A. (1977). Desensitization and self-control in the treatment of test anxiety. *Journal of Counseling Psychology, 24,* 272–280.

Dusek, J. B. (1980). The development of test anxiety in children. In I. G. Sarason (Ed.), *Test anxiety: Theory, research, and application* (pp. 87–110). Hilsdale, NJ: Erlbaum.

Feindler, E. L., & Fremouw, W. J. (1983). Stress inoculation training for adolescent anger problems. In D. Meichenbaum & M. E. Jaremko (Eds.), *Stress reduction and prevention* (pp. 451–486). New York: Plenum Press.

Flanders, J. P. (1968). A review of research on imitative behavior. *Psychological Bulletin, 69,* 316–337.

Glass, G. V., & Stanley, J. C. (1970). *Statistical methods in education and psychology.* Englewood Cliffs, NJ: Prentice-Hall.

Hussian, R. A., & Lawrence, P. S. (1978). The reduction of test, state, and trait anxiety by test specific and generalized stress inoculation training. *Cognitive Therapy and Research, 2,* 25–38.

Kerlinger, F. N., & Pedhazur, E. J. (1973). *Multiple regression in behavioral research.* New York: Holt, Rinehart & Winston.

Lent, R. W., & Rusell, R. K. (1978). Treatment of test anxiety by cue-controlled desensitization and study skills training. *Journal of Counseling Psychology, 25,* 217–224.

Mandler, G., & Sarason, S. B. (1952). A study of anxiety and learning. *Journal of Abnormal and Social Psychology, 47,* 166–173.

Mandler, G., & Sarason, S. B. (1953). The effect of prior experience and subjective failure on the evocation of test anxiety. *Journal of Personality, 21,* 336–341.

Meichenbaum, D. (1975). A self-instructional approach to stress management: A proposal for stress inoculation training. In C. D. Spielberger & I. G. Sarason (Eds.), *Stress and anxiety* (Vol. 1, pp. 237–263). New York: Hemisphere/Wiley.

Meichenbaum, D., & Cameron, R. (1983). Stress inoculation training: Toward a general paradigm for training coping skills. In D. Meichenbaum & M. E. Jaremko (Eds.), *Stress reduction and prevention* (pp. 115–154). New York: Plenum Press.

Meichenbaum, D., Turk, D., & Burstein, S. (1975). The nature of coping with stress. In C. D. Spielberger & I. G. Sarason (Eds.), *Stress and anxiety* (Vol. 2, pp. 337–360). New York: Hemisphere/Wiley.

Mitchell, K. R., & Ng, K. T. (1972). Effects of group counseling and behavior therapy on the academic achievement of test anxious students. *Journal of Counseling Psychology, 19,* 491–497.

Morris, L. W., & Liebert, R. M. (1970). Relationship of cognitive and emotional components of test anxiety to psychological arousal and academic performance. *Journal of Consulting and Clinical Psychology, 5,* 332–337.

Novaco, R. W. (1977). A stress inoculation approach to anger management in the training of law enforcement officers. *American Journal of Community Psychology, 21,* 285–290.

Novaco, R. W. (1979). The cognitive regulation of anger and stress. In P. L. Kendall & S. D. Hollon

(Eds.), *Cognitive-behavioral intervention: Theory, research, and procedures* (pp. 241–285). New York: Academic Press.

Rohrbaugh, J. B. (1979). *Women psychology's puzzle.* New York: Basic Books.

Sarason, I. G. (1960). Empirical findings and theoretical problems in the use of anxiety scales. *Psychological Bulletin, 57,* 403–415.

Sarason, I. G. (1972). Experimental approaches to test anxiety: Attention and the uses of information. In C. D. Spielberger (Ed.), *Anxiety: Current trends in theory and research* (Vol. 2, pp. 381–403) New York: Academic Press.

Sarason, I. G. (1975). Anxiety and self preoccupation. In C. D. Spielberger & I. G. Sarason (Eds.), *Stress and anxiety* (Vol. 2, pp. 27–43). Washington, DC: Hemisphere/Wiley.

Sarason, I. G. (1980). *Test anxiety: Theory, research, and application.* Hillsdale, NJ: Erlbaum.

Spielberger, C. D., Anton, W. D., & Bedell, J. (1976). The nature and treatment of test anxiety. In M. Zuckerman & C. D. Spielberger (Eds.), *Emotions and anxiety: New concepts, methods, and applications* (pp. 317–345). New York: Erlbaum/Wiley.

Spielberger, C. D., González, H. P., & Fletcher, T. (1979). *Test anxiety reduction, learning strategies, and academic performance.* In H. F. O'Neil, Jr., & C. D. Spielberger (Eds.), *Cognitive and affective learning strategies* (pp. 111–131). New York: Academic Press.

Spielberger, C. D., González, F., Martínez, A., Natalicio, L. F., & Natalicio, D. S. (1971). Development of the Spanish edition of the State–Trait Anxiety Inventory. *Interamerican Journal of Psychology, 5,* 145–158.

Spielberger, C. D., González, H. P., Taylor, C. J., Algaze, B., & Anton, W. D. (1978). Examination stress and test anxiety. In C. D. Spielberger & I. G. Sarason (Eds.). *Stress and anxiety* (Vol. 5, pp. 167–191). New York: Hemisphere/Wiley.

Suinn, R. M. (1969). The STABS, a measure of test anxiety for behavior therapy: Normative data. *Behavior, Research, and Therapy, 7,* 335–339.

Turk, D. (1976). *An expanded skills training approach for the treatment of experimentally induced pain.* Unpublished doctoral dissertation, University of Waterloo.

Veronen, L. J., & Kilpatrick, D. G. (1983). Stress management for rape victims. In D. Meichenbaum & M. E. Jaremko (Eds.), *Stress reduction and prevention* (pp. 341–374). New York: Plenum Press.

Wells, J. K., Howard, G. S., Nowlin, W. F., & Vargas, M. J. (1986). Presurgical anxiety and postsurgical pain and adjustment: Effects of a stress inoculation procedure. *Journal of Consulting and Clinical Psychology, 54,* 831–835.

Wine, J. D. (1971). Test anxiety and the direction of attention. *Psychological Bulletin, 76,* 92–104.

Wine, J. D. (1980). Cognitive-attentional theory of test anxiety. In I. G. Sarason (Ed.), *Test anxiety: Theory, research, and application* (pp. 349–385). Hillsdale, NJ: Erlbaum.

Wittmaier, B. C. (1972). Test anxiety and study habits. *Journal of Educational Research, 65,* 352–354.

III

CROSS-CULTURAL ASSESSMENT OF ANXIETY

12

Confirmatory Factor Analysis of the Test Anxiety Inventory

Jeri Benson and Elizabeth Tippets
University of Maryland, USA

Much research has been devoted to the study of test anxiety since this construct was introduced by Mandler and Sarason (1952) nearly 40 years ago. Decrements in achievement performance associated with high test anxiety have been of particular concern. To explain these decrements, recent test anxiety research has focused on cognitive-attentional theories (Wine, 1980). Sarason (1984), in particular, has commented on the importance of the cognitive-attentional approach in clarifying how test anxiety is experienced. Such explanations hold that, under stress, test-anxious individuals tend to worry about potential failure, and thus direct attention to themselves rather than focusing on the task at hand.

The measurement of test anxiety has been advanced by the conceptualization of worry and emotionality as separate components of the construct (Deffenbacher, 1980; Liebert & Morris, 1967; Schwarzer, 1984). Emotionality refers to the feelings and the physiological (autonomic) arousal experienced by examinees during testing. Measures of worry assess the cognitive concerns that examinees may have about their performance during testing. However, only the worry component has been found to be consistently associated with decreased performance (Deffenbacher, 1977; Hodapp, 1982; Holroyd, Westbrook, Wolf, & Badhorn, 1978; Morris & Liebert, 1970; O'Neil, Judd, & Hedl, 1977; Spielberger, 1980).

In a study by Morris and Liebert (1970), self-report measures of test anxiety correlated only .34 with physical measurements of autonomic arousal. Therefore, it seems likely that the perception of emotionality, not autonomic arousal per se, is measured by emotionality scales. Moreover, because correlations between self-report measures of worry and emotionality have varied between .55–.76 in various studies (Deffenbacher, 1980), it would seem that measures of both constructs assess, to some degree, cognitive behaviors that interfere with achievement performance.

Although there are many good instruments for assessing test anxiety, most do not provide separate measures of worry and emotionality (Schwarzer, 1984). An exception is the Test Anxiety Inventory (TAI; Spielberger, Gonzalez, Taylor, Algaze, & Anton, 1978), which contains factorially derived measures of these two components. The TAI has been adapted and used extensively by researchers in a number of countries, for example, Hagtvet (1984) in Norway, Schwarzer, Jerusalem, & Lange (1982) in Germany, and van der Ploeg (1982) in The Netherlands.

The TAI Manual (Spielberger, 1980) provides separate normative information for male and female subjects. Moreover, in research studies of the TAI, it is common practice to take gender into account in analyzing the data and reporting the results. The rationale for this practice is that the mean test anxiety scores for female subjects are consistently somewhat higher than those for male subjects. Nevertheless, it is tacitly assumed that the scores for male and female subjects have the same meaning (i.e., the underlying structure of the scale is the same for both sexes).

In a study of the factor structure of the German TAI, based on a sample of 1,848 sixth- and ninth-grade students, Schwarzer (1984) used the data for the girls in the sample to explore the factor structure of the scale, and the male sample for replication. The Emotionality and Worry factors that were identified for both sexes correlated .67 for the girls and .54 for the boys. Moreover, the loadings for girls on these factors were consistently higher than those for boys. Although the possibility that these differences were due to chance was not tested, Schwarzer concluded that the possibility that the TAI's structure may be different for boys and girls needed further research.

Van der Ploeg (1982) factored the TAI item responses of Dutch medical school students separately for men and women, and also found gender differences. Similarly, Hedl (1984) analyzed the TAI data separately for a large sample of American undergraduates and found differences in the item loadings for men and women. However, when the factor solutions were evaluated for invariance it was concluded that the similarity of the factor axes was very strong.

Given the inconsistencies with regard to gender differences in previous factor studies of the TAI, the question arises as to whether the TAI scores of male and female subjects have the same meaning. Put differently, does the TAI measure the same construct to the same degree for both male and female subjects? Thus, the essential measurement issue in question is factor structure invariance.

The present study responds to Schwarzer's (1984) explicit call for research on gender differences in the TAI by testing the invariance of the TAI factor structure for men and women. Through confirmatory factor analysis, using maximum likelihood estimation, the appropriateness of a two-factor structure for both sexes is evaluated, and whether the item loadings, item errors, and factor correlations are the same for both sexes is determined. Each of these possibilities (or hypotheses) was tested by comparing the fit of a succession of increasingly restricted models according to methods outlined by Jöreskog (1971) and Bentler and Bonett (1980). In this type of analysis, the individual items are considered to be indicators of the latent factors they represent.

METHOD AND PROCEDURES

Sample

The sample consisted of 572 undergraduate and graduate students who were enrolled in three different educational measurement and statistics courses. Boomsma (1982) recommended that sample sizes of at least 200 be used in confirmatory factor analysis studies, and he has demonstrated that sample size may influence various fit indices. Therefore, it was decided to use equal numbers of men and women, drawn from a total of 711 available cases, for whom there were no missing data. All 286 men in the sample were used. A random sample of 286 women was drawn, using the SPSS-X sample selection procedure (McGraw-Hill, 1983). The mean age for the total sample was 27; the mean ages of the men and women were 25 and 29, respectively.

Test Anxiety Inventory

The TAI consists of 20 items presented in a Likert-style format with four ordered categories (Spielberger, 1980). A series of factor analyses was used in the development of the TAI and in subsequent studies of the English form and adaptations in other languages. The investigations have established a two-factor structure for the TAI, composed of correlated Worry and Emotionality factors. As reported in the TAI Manual (Spielberger, 1980), 16 of the 20 items have loadings on either Worry or Emotionality, but not on both factors. The 8 items that constitute the TAI Worry subscale are Items 3, 4, 5, 6, 7, 14, 17, and 20; the 8 items that form the Emotionality subscale are Items 2, 8, 9, 10, 11, 15, 16, and 18. The TAI total scale and both subscales have been shown to have high internal consistency reliability in previous research. These findings were confirmed in the present study: Cronbach's alpha for the full scale was .92; the alphas for the Worry and Emotionality subscales were .89 and .87, respectively.

Procedures

The data were collected in two different semesters in the context of a study of test anxiety (Benson, 1987). The TAI was administered as part of the questionnaire developed for that study, using the standard directions as reported in the TAI Manual (Spielberger, 1980). As the two-factor structure of the TAI has been well documented in the literature, it was decided to test the two-factor model, using only the 16 TAI items in the Worry and Emotionality subscales. The four items that were omitted from the present analysis were not used in computing scores on the Worry and Emotionality subscales because double loadings on these items are reported in the TAI Manual. The following four hierarchical models were tested:

- Model 1 assumed that a two-factor structure was appropriate for both men and women.
- Model 2 assumed both a two-factor structure and that item loadings were the same for both sexes.
- Model 3 assumed a two-factor structure, equal item loadings, and equal item errors (uniquenesses) for both sexes.
- Model 4 assumed a two-factor structure, equal loadings, equal item errors, and equal factor correlations for both sexes.

In evaluating the fit of each of the four models, assuming that a two-factor structure was appropriate for both sexes, the test of the difference between Model 1 and Model 2 evaluates whether the factor loadings (i.e., the factor patterns) are the same for men and women. The difference between Model 2 and Model 3 tests whether the item errors are the same for men and women, given that the factor loadings are the same for both sexes. The difference between Model 3 and Model

4 tests whether the factor correlations are the same for men and women, given that the loadings and errors are the same for both groups.

The factor analyses were performed, using covariance matrices in which each item was constrained to load only on the factor with which it correlated the highest, as reported in the TAI Manual. Parameter estimates and model fit statistics were obtained, using LISREL VII (Jöreskog & Sörbom, 1988). Confirmatory factor analyses of the four models were performed following Jöreskog's (1971) approach to testing the invariance of factor structure simultaneously across groups.

The four models were hierarchical in the sense that each successive model was more restrictive than the one that preceded it. Moreover, each model was associated with a question of theoretical and psychometric interest relating to the comparability of the factor structure for men and women. As the models were tested, a chi-square goodness-of-fit statistic evaluated the point at which the scale was no longer invariant for men and women.

RESULTS

The means and standard deviations of the scores of men, women, and the total sample on the 16-team TAI and on the 8-item Worry and Emotionality subscales are reported in Table 1. To permit comparison with previous studies, the means and standard deviations of the total scores for the 20-item TAI are also reported. Separate t tests were run for men and women for the TAI total scores and for each subscale. Significant differences ($p < .05$) between men and women were noted for the 16-item and 20-item TAIs and for the Emotionality subscale, with women scoring higher than men in each comparison.

The results of the simultaneous confirmatory factor analyses of the 16-item scale for the four models, tested across men and women, are presented in Table 2. The chi-square values for these tests tend to be inflated for two reasons: the large sample size and the use of Pearson correlation coefficients with four ordered categories. Therefore, the goodness of fit of the models must be judged according to several additional indices. Accordingly, the ratios of chi-square to degrees of freedom (χ_2/df), the goodness-of-fit index (GFI), and the root mean square residual (RMR) are also presented in Table 2.

For acceptable fit, the chi-square ratio should be less than 3 (Carmines & McIver, 1981). The GFI is an index obtained from the LISREL program that mea-

Table 1   Means and Standard Deviations for the 20- and 16-Item Test Anxiety Inventory (TAI) and the Emotionality and Worry Subscales

Scale	Men (n = 286)		Women (n = 286)		Total sample	
	M	SD	M	SD	M	SD
16-item TAI	29.16	8.60	31.56	9.97	30.36	9.38
Emotionality	15.88	5.05	17.91	5.91	16.89	5.59
Worry	13.28	4.28	13.65	4.84	13.47	4.55
20-item TAI	37.32	9.97	40.03	11.48	38.67	10.82

Note. The means and standard deviations for the Emotionality and Worry subscales were based on eight items each.

Table 2 Results of Simultaneous Confirmatory Factor Analysis for 16-Item Scale

Model and description	χ^2	df	χ^2/df	GFI		RMR	
				Men	Women	Men	Women
Model 1							
Equal number of factors	483	206	2.34	.89	.90	.03	.03
Model 2							
Equal number of factors	495	220	2.25	.89	.90	.03	.04
Equal loadings							
Model 3							
Equal number of factors	520	236	2.20	.88	.90	.04	.04
Equal loadings							
Equal errors							
Model 4							
Equal number of factors	531	239	2.22	.88	.90	.07	.07
Equal loadings							
Equal errors							
Equal factor correlations							

Model comparisons	χ^2	df
Model 1 vs. Model 2	12	14
Model 2 vs. Model 3	25	16
Model 3 vs. Model 4	11	3[a]

Note. GFI = goodness-of-fit index, RMR = root mean square residual.
[a]Critical value chi-square difference (3) = 7.81 ($p < .05$).

sures the relative amount of variances and covariances jointly accounted for by the model. For acceptable fit, the GFI should be close to 1.0. The RMR, which is the average of the residual variances and covariances, should be close to zero if the model fits well.

The GFI and RMR are reported in Table 2 for both the male and the female samples; LISREL fits the model to each group separately, then provides a chi-square statistic of overall model–data fit. The chi-square values shown in Table 2 were all significant (which is expected with large samples); the chi-square ratios were all close to 2.0; the GFI ranged from .88 to .90; and the RMR ranged from .03 to .07. Thus, all four indices indicated an acceptable fit of the separate models.

The next question that was examined was that of parsimony. Model comparisons were made to determine at which point the 16-item TAI was no longer invariant for men and women. The model comparisons are shown in the lower part of Table 2. The first two chi-square difference tests were not significant. However, the comparison of Model 4 to Model 3 was significant (χ^2 difference = 11.0, $p < .05$). Taken together, the model comparison difference tests indicated that a two-factor structure fit the data well, and that the item loadings and item errors were the same for men and women. However, the correlation among the latent factors was different for men and women. Although the test of the additional restriction of equal factor correlations was statistically significant, this difference is of little practical importance; the correlation among the latent factors in Model 3 was .816 for men and .813 for women.

Estimates of the item loadings for Model 4 are presented in Table 3. All of the loadings were .40 or higher and were statistically significant ($p < .05$). The

Table 3 Item Loadings For the 16-Item Scale
Based on Model 4

	Subscales	
Item	Emotionality	Worry
2	.58	
8	.66	
9	.70	
10	.56	
11	.70	
15	.73	
16	.70	
18	.55	
3		.58
4		.57
5		.40
6		.41
7		.60
14		.57
17		.57
20		.58

Note. Items that were not allowed to load on the
Emotionality and Worry factors are blank.

median item loadings for the Worry and Emotionality factors were .57 and .68, respectively. The observed correlations between the Worry and Emotionality subscales for the 16-item TAI were .70 for men and .72 for women. However, the correlation between the latent Worry and Emotionality factors for Model 4 (the most restrictive and parsimonious model) was .814 for both men and women for the 16-item scale. The small difference in the magnitudes of the subscale and latent factor correlations is attributable to the fact that the subscale correlation reflects the error contained in the observed subscale scores, whereas the correlation between the latent factors is independent of measurement error.

DISCUSSION AND CONCLUSIONS

The findings in the present study that the number of factors, loadings, and errors were the same for men and women is encouraging. The finding of unequal correlations among the latent factors was primarily influenced by the large sample size, as the correlation between the two factors was highly similar for men and women (.816 and .813, respectively). It may therefore be concluded that the 16 items that constitute the TAI Worry and Emotionality subscales have the same meaning for men and women, and that there was no evidence that the items were biased in terms of gender. The findings also provide strong evidence that the latent construct of test anxiety, as defined by the 16 TAI items, is measured similarly for men and women.

For the present study, the mean scores on the 8-item Worry and Emotionality subscales were similar to those obtained from the college-age samples used in the development of the original English version of the TAI. However, the correlations between the subscales in this study were higher than those typically reported in the literature. The higher correlation might be attributed to the relatively higher age and greater heterogeneity of the current sample as compared with other studies. The sample in this study, which included both undergraduate and graduate students from a variety of academic disciplines, was considerably more diverse than those used in other studies.

In studies of the factor structure of the TAI, previous researchers have concluded that there were differences in the pattern of loadings for men and women (Schwarzer, 1984; van der Ploeg, 1982). The results of the present confirmatory factor analysis of the 16-item TAI revealed a similar two-factor pattern for men and women, along with demonstrated equality of the factor loadings and item errors. The only statistically significant finding was in the correlation between the latent factors. However, this very small difference was of no practical significance.

The discrepancies between the findings of this study and those of Schwarzer (1984) and van der Ploeg (1982) may be due to (a) differences in the populations (they studied grade-school children and medical students, respectively), (b) differences in methodology (exploratory factor analysis vs. different approaches to confirmatory factor analysis, and (c) cultural differences (American, German, and Dutch). In a study of subjects similar in age to those in the present study, Hedl (1984) noted differences in item loadings for men and women, but concluded that there were no differences between the factor axes. A similar conclusion may be drawn from the findings of the present study.

REFERENCES

Benson, J. (July 1987). *Causal components of statistical test anxiety in adults: An exploratory study.* Paper presented at the Eighth Annual Society for Test Anxiety Research, Bergen, Norway.

Bentler, P., & Bonett, D. (1980). Significance tests and goodness of fit in the analysis of covariance structures. *Psychological Bulletin, 88,* 588–606.

Boomsma, A. (1982). *The robustness of LISREL against small sample sizes in factor analysis models.* In K. G. Jöreskog & T. Wold (Eds.), Systems under indirect observation: Causality, structure, prediction (Part 1, pp. 149–173). Amsterdam: North-Holland.

Carmines, E., & McIver, J. (1981). Analyzing models with unobserved variables: Analysis of covariance structures. In G. W. Bohrnstedt & E. F. Borgotta (Eds.), *Sociological measurement: Current issues* (pp. 65–115). Beverly Hills, CA: Sage.

Deffenbacher, J. L. (1977). Relationship of worry and emotionality to performance on the Miller Analogies Test. *Journal of Educational Psychology, 69,* 191–195.

Deffenbacher, J. L. (1980). Worry and emotionality in test anxiety. In I. G. Sarason (Ed.), *Test anxiety* (pp. 111–128). Hillsdale, NJ: Erlbaum.

Hagtvet, K. A. (1984). A Norwegian adaptation of the TAI: A first tryout. *International Review of Applied Psychology, 33,* 257–265.

Hedl, J. J. (1984). A factor analytic study of the Test Anxiety Inventory. *International Review of Applied Psychology, 33,* 267–283.

Hodapp. V. (1982). Causal inference from nonexperimental research on anxiety and educational achievement. In H. W. Krohne & L. Laux (Eds.), *Achievement, stress and anxiety* (pp. 355–372). Washington, DC: Hemisphere.

Holroyd, K. A., Westbrook, T., Wolf, M., & Badhorn, E. (1978). Performance, cognition, and psychological responding in test anxiety. *Journal of Abnormal Psychology, 87,* 442–451.

Jöreskog, K. G. (1971). Simultaneous factor analysis in several populations. *Psychometrika, 36,* 409–426.

Jöreskog, K. G., & Sörbom, D. (1988). *LISREL VII: A guide to the program and applications.* Mooresville, IN: Scientific Software.

Liebert, R. M., & Morris, L. W. (1967). Cognitive and emotional components of test anxiety: A distinction and some initial data. *Psychological Reports, 20,* 975-978.

Mandler, G., & Sarason, S. B. (1952). A study of anxiety and learning. *Journal of Abnormal and Social Psychology, 47,* 166-173.

McGraw-Hill (1983). *SPSS-X user's guide.* New York: Author.

Morris, L. W., & Liebert, L. M. (1970). Relationship of cognitive and emotional components of test anxiety to physiological arousal and academic performance. *Journal of Consulting and Clinical Psychology, 35,* 332-337.

O'Neil, H. F, Jr., Judd, W. A., & Hedl, J. J., Jr. (1977). State anxiety and performance in computer-based learning environments. In J. E. Sieber, H. F. O'Neil, Jr., & S. Tobias (Eds.), *Anxiety, learning and instruction.* Hillsdale, NJ: Erlbaum.

Sarason, S. B. (1984). Stress, anxiety, and cognitive interference: Reactions to tests. *Journal of Personality and Social Psychology, 46,* 929-938.

Schwarzer, R. (1984). Worry and emotionality as separate components in test anxiety. *International Review of Applied Psychology, 33,* 205-220.

Schwarzer, R., Jerusalem, M., & Lange, B. (1982) A longitudinal study of worry and emotionality in German secondary school children. In R. Schwarzer, H. M. van der Ploeg, & C. D. Spielberger (Eds.), *Advances in test anxiety research* (Vol. 1, pp. 67-81). Lisse, The Netherlands: Swets & Zeitlinger B. V.

Spielberger, C. D. (1980). *Preliminary professional manual for the Test Anxiety Inventory.* Palo Alto, CA: Consulting Psychologists Press.

Spielberger, C. D., Gonzalez, H. P., Taylor, C. J., Algaze, B., & Anton, W. D. (1978). Examination stress and test anxiety. In C. D. Spielberger & I. G. Sarason (Eds.), *Stress and anxiety* (Vol. 5, pp. 167-191). New York: Hemisphere/Wiley.

Van der Ploeg, H. M. (1982). The relationship of worry and emotionality to performance in Dutch school children. In R. Schwarzer, H. M. van der Ploeg, & C. D. Spielberger (Eds.), *Advances in test anxiety research* (Vol. 1, pp. 55-66). The Netherlands: Swets & Zeitlinger B. V.

Wine, J. D. (1980). Cognitive-attentional theory of test anxiety. In I. G. Sarason (Ed.), *Test anxiety: Theory, research, and applications* (pp. 349-384). Hillsdale, NJ: Erlbaum.

13

A Decade of Research
on State–Trait Anxiety in Brazil

Angela M. B. Biaggio
Universidade Federal do Rio Grande do Sul, Porto Alegre, Brazil

This chapter describes findings based on a decade of research on state and trait anxiety in Brazil. The following points, stimulated by Spielberger's (1966, 1972) work on anxiety, were addressed in this research: (a) evaluation of the distinction between anxiety as a transitory emotional state (S-Anxiety) and individual differences in anxiety as a stable personality trait (T-Anxiety); (b) development of Portuguese measures of state and trait anxiety with adequate psychometric properties, and (c) the applicability of these measures for cross-cultural research in Brazil.

Spielberger's State–Trait Anxiety Inventory (STAI; Spielberger, Gorsuch, & Lushene, 1970) had already been translated and adapted in more than a dozen languages at the time this research was initiated. The first step in this research program was adapting the STAI for use in the Brazilian and Portuguese cultures. A Portuguese children's form was also constructed. Both of these scales were then used to investigate a number of problems of diverse theoretical interest that are described in this chapter.

DEVELOPMENT OF THE PORTUGUESE FORMS
OF THE STAI

Translations of the individual STAI items by Biaggio and Natalicio (1979) were evaluated by expert judges, and minor reformulations were made. The preliminary Portuguese STAI, consisting of 24 S-Anxiety and 22 T-Anxiety items, were then administered to four samples of Portuguese–English bilingual college students. The English STAI was administered to these students, with a 1-week test–retest interval, except in one of the samples in which the students took both forms on the same day. To control for possible order effects, half of the subjects in each sample were given the English form first, followed by the preliminary Portuguese form; the other half were given the Portuguese form first.

In selecting the final set of 20 S-Anxiety and 20 T-Anxiety items for the experimental Portuguese form of the STAI, the data for the four independent samples

The research reported in this article is restricted to studies conducted in Brazil by the author and her students. Angela M. B. Biaggio is professor of psychology and education at the Federal University of Rio Grande do Sul, Porto Alegre, Brazil, and Senior Researcher of the Brazilian National Research Council.

were combined and item-remainder correlations for men and women were computed. The selection of the final set of items for the experimental Portuguese STAI was based on these item-remainder correlations and on the correlations between the scores on each preliminary Portuguese item and the corresponding English STAI item. The psychometric characteristics of the experimental Portuguese STAI have been reported in detail by Biaggio, Natalicio, and Spielberger (1976). The T-Anxiety means for male and female Brazilian college students and the mean S-Anxiety score for Brazilian women were slightly higher than those for U.S. students (Spielberger et al., 1970). In contrast, the mean S-Anxiety score for Brazilian men was slightly lower than that for U.S. undergraduates. Alpha coefficients calculated by using the Kuder–Richardson 20, as modified by Chronbach (1951), were .75 or higher for the Portuguese S-Anxiety and T-Anxiety scales for both men and women.

The median item-remainder correlation for the Portuguese S-Anxiety Scale was .59 for men and .62 for women. These item-remainder correlations were .50 or higher for 17 of the 20 S-Anxiety items, and .30 or higher for all but one of these items. The T-Anxiety item-remainder correlations were even higher than those obtained for the S-Anxiety scale for both men and women. With but a single exception, the item-remainder correlations for the T-Anxiety items were .40 or higher; the median item-remainder correlations for men and women were .75 and .60, respectively.

The equivalence of the experimental Portuguese STAI and the English STAI was determined by computing correlations between scores on the two S-Anxiety and T-Anxiety scales for each of the four bilingual samples, and for the data from all samples combined. The values of these correlations for the combined data were .69 for S-Anxiety, .77 for T-Anxiety, and .90 and .95, respectively, for the sample who took both tests on the same day. These values were slightly lower for the other three samples, which would be expected as a function of the 1-week test–retest interval that introduced an additional source of unreliability.

The construct validity of the Portuguese STAI was evaluated in several investigations in which the S-Anxiety and T-Anxiety scales were administered under stressful and nonstressful conditions. In one study, the two scales were administered to 17 college students immediately before a statistics examination, and were subsequently readministered during a regular class period. The preexamination S-Anxiety mean score (45.71) was more than 10 points higher than in the nonstressful condition (35.35); this difference was highly significant ($t = 3.32, p < .005$). In contrast, the T-Anxiety means were essentially the same in the stressful ($M = 37.53$) and nonstressful ($M = 37.35$) experimental conditions. These results demonstrated that scores on the Portuguese S-Anxiety Scale increased in response to situational stress, whereas the T-Anxiety Scale was relatively impervious to situational factors. Similar findings have been reported in investigations of examination stress in which the English STAI was used (Spielberger et al., 1970).

Further evidence of the Portuguese STAI's construct validity was demonstrated in a study by Kacelnik, Oliveira, and Farias (1975). These investigators tested 30 eighth-grade students in an experimental situation in which cognitive dissonance was induced. The students were required to write arguments in favor of having to take an unexpected, very difficult exam under low-reward conditions. The students' scores on the Portuguese STAI S-Anxiety and T-Anxiety scales on this occasion were then compared with their scores in a neutral condition. The S-

Anxiety scores were substantially higher after dissonance induction (t = 6.78, p < .001), whereas T-Anxiety scores were essentially the same in the dissonance and neutral situations (t = .58).

Taruma, Fernandez, and Paschoal (1975) found significantly higher S-Anxiety scores 24 hr before patients underwent minor surgery than when the same patients were discharged from the hospital (t = 5.89, p < .001). In contrast, the difference in T-Anxiety scores before and after surgery was not statistically significant. Similar findings with regard to the affects of imminent surgery on scores on the English STAI have been reported by a number of investigators (e.g., Spielberger, Auerbach, Wadsworth, Dunn, & Taulbee, 1973).

The Portuguese Language Form of the STAIC

A test-construction procedure analogous to that described earlier was followed in developing the Portuguese form of the State–Trait Anxiety Inventory for Children (STAIC; Spielberger, 1973). A preliminary translation of the STAIC items was evaluated by five Portuguese–English bilingual psychologists and one translator-interpreter, and their suggestions were taken into consideration in revising the items. The preliminary Portuguese STAIC items were then given to 50 bilingual fourth-, fifth-, and sixth-grade children enrolled in an American, Catholic school in Rio de Janeiro. The test was given twice, once in English and once in Portuguese, with a 2-week test–retest interval. The correlations between the two forms of the STAI were .42 for the S-Anxiety Scale and .60 for the T-Anxiety Scale.

The internal consistency of the Portuguese STAIC was checked with a sample of 54 nonbilingual Brazilian children. Alpha correlations of .63 and .56 were obtained for the S-Anxiety and T-Anxiety scales, respectively. The item-remainder values for the S-Anxiety and T-Anxiety items were also satisfactory, although somewhat lower than those obtained for the adult form. Test–retest correlations were .66 for S-Anxiety and .73 for T-Anxiety, indicating satisfactory temporal stability.

Concurrent and construct validity of the Portuguese STAIC was verified in several different ways. Children's scores on the T-Anxiety Scale of the Portuguese STAIC correlated significantly with teachers' ratings of the children's anxiety (r = .61, p < .01). In a second study, anxiety was measured in a dentist's waiting room, and higher S-Anxiety scores were found, providing evidence for the construct validity of the S-Anxiety Scale. In another study, children took the Portuguese STAIC shortly before a mathematics examination, and the scale was readministered during a nonstressful regular class period. Contrary to expectation, however, no increase in S-Anxiety was observed in the examination situation. This finding leads to the speculation that modern pedagogy in Brazil, at least in the school where this study took place, has decreased "number fright."

The translation and adaptation of the Portuguese STAIC has been described in detail by Biaggio (1980). Norms for the adults and the children's forms are reported in the manuals for the Portuguese forms (Biaggio & Natalicio, 1979; Biaggio, 1983) in terms of percentiles and McCall's T scores (M = 50, SD = 10). The norms for the adult form are based on the scores of 1,843 university and high-school students from Rio de Janeiro and Santos (Sao Paulo). The norms for the children's form were based on the scores of 842 children from public and private schools in Rio de Janeiro. Once the Portuguese forms of the STAI and the STAIC were considered adequate for use with Brazilian subjects, a number of experiments were conducted to test hypotheses of theoretical interest. The findings in these investigations are reported in the following section.

RESEARCH WITH THE PORTUGUESE STAI
AND STAIC

Anxiety and Locus of Control

The relation between anxiety and locus of control, one of the central constructs in Rotter's (1966, 1975) social learning theory, was investigated in two studies (Biaggio, 1985). Rotter postulated that the effect of reinforcement on behavior depends, in part, on the perception of whether reinforcement is contingent on, or independent of, a person's behavior. Reinforcement in certain situations, for example, a game of dice, in which reinforcement depends on chance strengthens a belief in external control. In other situations, such as solving a mathematical problem, where success depends on ability, reinforcement leads to a belief in internal control. A person's cumulative reinforcement history contributes to generalized expectancies that are expressed as tendencies toward an internal or external locus of control.

The goal of the first investigation was to clarify the nature of the relation between anxiety and locus of control by bringing the state–trait distinction to bear on the problem (Biaggio, 1985). Most studies in the locus-of-control literature (Lefcourt, 1976) have reported positive correlations between anxiety and externality, and have used measures of trait anxiety rather than state anxiety as these concepts are defined by Spielberger. However, except for studies by Jolley and Spielberger (1973) and Archer (1979), little attention seems to have been given to the distinction between state and trait anxiety.

On the basis of previous research, externality was expected to correlate positively with T-Anxiety. It was also predicted that internal subjects would show more S-Anxiety than external subjects in "luck" situations, whereas external subjects would show more S-Anxiety in "ability" situations. The subjects were 86 female psychology students, between 16–25 years of age, enrolled in a Brazilian university. They reported individually to the laboratory to participate in the experiment and responded to the following measures: (a) the Portuguese version of Rotter's Internal–External Locus of Control Scale developed by Soares (1977), who presents acceptable data on reliability; and (b) the Portuguese form of the STAI.

Each subject was classified on the basis of her locus-of-control scores as predominantly internal or external. Internals (scores $\geq$ 10) and externals (scores $\geq$ 15) were randomly assigned to either luck or ability experimental conditions, which are now described.

Luck Condition

Subjects were asked to engage in a card-guessing game in which two sets of 10 cards were used. The experimenter placed one card at a time face down on the table, and the subject tried to match it, taking one card from her own set. Subjects were told that getting it right was a matter of luck.

Ability Condition

Each subject was asked to solve an apparently easy puzzle, consisting of 15 pieces to be fitted into a frame. The task, which was in fact rather difficult, was presented as a test of space perception that supposedly correlated highly with general intelligence. Subjects were told they would have 10 min to solve it.

The STAI was administered to each subject immediately after the completion of the experimental task. The correlation between T-Anxiety and externality was .47 ($p < .05$); the S-Anxiety–externality correlation was .22, which was not significant. The T-Anxiety–externality correlation and the results of the analysis of variance (ANOVA) of T-Anxiety scores were consistent with the hypothesis that externals would score significantly higher than internals ($F = 6.21$, $p < .05$). The ANOVA results for S-Anxiety did not reach statistical significance.

The data for T-Anxiety confirmed the hypotheses that externals have higher scores on this variable, regardless of the nature of the task. Although the findings replicate the results of previous studies in different cultures, the relation between S-Anxiety and locus of control was still unclear. The externals were slightly higher than the internals on S-Anxiety in the ability situation, but this difference was not significant, and the means for externals and internals were practically the same in the luck situation. Although the statistical analysis of S-Anxiety scores did not reach significance, the experimental manipulation nevertheless appears to have had some effect; otherwise externals would have been more anxious in the luck situation, as was found for T-Anxiety.

In a second experiment (Biaggio, 1985), the experimental design was analogous to the first study, but children served as subjects. An incentive variable was also added because it was felt that the luck versus ability experimental manipulation was not very powerful because of the inconsequentiality of not doing well in the laboratory setting. It was predicted in this study that the incentive condition would lead to higher S-Anxiety than would the nonincentive condition. Additionally, it was expected that internality would increase with age (or school grade), as was found in Israel by Milgram (1971).

The subjects were 56 fourth-, fifth-, and sixth-grade children (36 girls and 20 boys) from a private school in Rio de Janeiro. The children, ranging in age from $9^{1}/_{2}$ to 13 years, were chosen on the basis of their scores on the Portuguese version of Milgram and Milgram's (1975) Locus of Control Scale for Children, as adapted by Feres (1982). As Feres (1982) found no significant sex differences among Brazilian children on this measure, gender was not an independent variable in the study's design.

Internal- and external-locus-of-control children were randomly assigned to one of the following four experimental conditions: luck with incentive, luck without incentive, ability with incentive, and ability without incentive. The luck versus ability variable was manipulated in the same way as in the previous experiment, with the same instructions and materials. In the incentive condition, the children were told that whoever solved the puzzle in the least amount of time (ability condition), or whoever guessed the highest number of cards (luck condition), would receive a prize (a large, attractively wrapped box placed on a shelf in the experimental room). In the nonincentive condition, the children were told nothing about prizes, and the box was not in the room. Each student was tested individually. After the experimental manipulation, each child took the Portuguese STAIC.

To minimize communication among the children, one grade was tested at a time.

The effect of externality–internality on S-Anxiety was highly significant, with externals showing higher S-Anxiety than internals, regardless of their experimental condition. The incentive manipulation was also highly significant, revealing higher S-Anxiety in the incentive condition, regardless of internality–externality or the luck versus ability experimental condition. However, the prediction of a positive correlation between externality and T-Anxiety was not confirmed. In fact, a strong negative correlation ($r = .68$, $p < .005$) between these variables was found. The internals in all four experimental conditions had higher T-Anxiety scores than the externals. Surprisingly, there was no correlation between S-Anxiety and T-Anxiety ($r = .08$.). When measured in adults under neutral conditions, these two aspects of anxiety generally correlate in the .60s.

In the children's study, externality and incentive accounted for most of the variance in S-Anxiety. It is possible that external children are more prone to situational (state) anxiety and that external reinforcement may be needed to mobilize this anxiety. Perhaps children are only affected by intrinsic motivation (implicit in our ego-involving instructions) as they get older. Ideally, longitudinal studies would be more appropriate to investigate this kind of problem, as was suggested by Steitz (1982).

Differences in the instruments used with children and adults, plus the peculiarities of the results for the children in the second study, make the findings of the two studies difficult to integrate. The most obvious conclusion is that relations between locus of control and state or trait anxiety appear to be different for children than for adults. Findings such as the significant positive correlation between T-Anxiety and externality, and increasing internality with age, are of interest because they replicate similar findings in a different culture.

On the basis of the findings in the two anxiety–locus-of-control studies, it was concluded that the relation between these variables may be different for adults and children. Although one can only speculate at this point, there may be fewer demands on Brazilian university students than on Brazilian children, and consequently less anxiety about performance among Brazilian university students than in other countries. Moreover, as internality correlates positively with school achievement (Feres, 1982), it seems reasonable that pressures from parents and school authorities may lead the internal child to become more anxious about achievement in both luck- and ability-dependent situations, whereas college students may be less vulnerable to such pressures because they are less dependent on parental approval.

Anxiety and Moral Judgment

The objective of this study was to investigate the relation between maturity of moral judgment and state and trait anxiety (Biaggio, 1990, in press). Kohlberg's (1963, 1981) theory of moral judgment, which arises from the cognitive-development constructivist paradigm proposed by Piaget, occupies a prominent place in current developmental psychology, especially the study of moral development. According to Kohlberg, maturity of moral judgment evolves through an invariant sequence of stages that parallel Piaget's stages of cognitive development.

In the classic study in this area, preadolescents participated in group discussions with the objective of raising their stage of moral judgment (Blatt & Kohlberg, 1975). Gains were significant in comparison to control groups.

In Kohlberg's (1963, 1981) theory, the principle that accounts for progression to higher stages is that of cognitive conflict (Turiel, 1969), a concept akin to Piaget's notion of disequilibrium. Exposure to moral dilemmas one stage above one's own stimulates upward change. Although widely accepted, Kohlberg's theory has not escaped criticism. One major criticism is that Kohlberg (as well as Piaget) overemphasized cognition and minimized the role of affect. In keeping with this criticism, Biaggio (1967) found that moral judgment correlated with guilt feelings. Consequently, she argued that correlations of moral judgment with moral behavior are mediated by personality variables such as ego control.

The objective of this study was to examine relation between the cognitive and affective aspects of moral development by investigating the links between anxiety and the maturity of moral judgment. The following hypotheses were tested: (a) Participation in moral judgment discussion groups will increase S-Anxiety, and (b) T-Anxiety will correlate negatively with maturity of moral judgment. On the assumption that cognition and affect are inseparable, the rationale for the first hypothesis is that cognitive conflict is likely to generate an emotional reaction. Regarding the second hypothesis, because anxiety is generally considered a nonadaptive, disruptive trait, it should correlate negatively with desirable characteristics such as intelligence, learning, and moral judgment.

The subjects in this study were 14- to 16-year-old 10th-graders from a public school in Porto Alegre, Brazil. The experimental group consisted of 24 subjects (8 boys and 16 girls); the control group consisted of 20 subjects (10 boys and 10 girls). The data were collected in three sessions, with a 1-week interval between sessions. In the first session, the subjects were pretested on moral judgment, as measured by the Differential Issues Test (DIT; Rest, 1976) as adapted by Bzuneck (1979).

Before the second session, the students were randomly assigned to the experimental and control conditions. The experimental group was further divided into two subgroups ($n = 12$) in order to ensure an adequate and manageable number of students for the moral dilemma discussions. In assigning students to these subgroups, their moral judgment pretest scores were taken into account so that there would be a wide variance within each group in order to foster different stage thinking during the discussions.

During the second session, one of Blatt and Kohlberg's (1975) dilemmas was used for the group discussion, which was led by the researcher in one group and by an experienced graduate student in the other. Subjects in the control group engaged in a placebo activity that consisted of taking the Portuguese version of a self-concept scale. Following the discussion, all subjects took the STAI.

For the statistical analysis, the data for the two experimental groups were combined. The mean S-Anxiety score of the girls was significantly higher in the experimental session ($M = 42.06$) than in the posttest session ($M = 38.13$); the S-Anxiety mean for the experimental group was also significantly higher than the corresponding mean for the control group ($M = 38.00$). In addition, gains in moral maturity attributable to the discussion were negatively correlated with S-Anxiety for boys ($r = .78, p < .001$). Although the corresponding correlation for the girls was also negative, it did not reach significance.

The second hypothesis was tested by correlating the DIT and T-Anxiety scores. These correlations were negative as predicted, but reached significance only for the boys (raw scores: $r = .69, p < .001$; T scores: $r = .48, p < .02$). Thus, S-Anxiety was consistently higher during the session in which there was discussion of moral dilemmas than it was when no such discussion occurred, and maturity of moral judgment was negatively related to trait anxiety, but only for boys.

The theoretical relevance of the confirmation of the first hypothesis provides evidence of a relation between the cognitive and emotional aspects of morality, and justifies the criticism of Kohlberg (1963) for ignoring the emotional aspects of morality. In essence, our findings indicated that cognitive conflict as conceptualized by Kohlberg was related to S-Anxiety as conceptualized by Spielberger (1966).

Regarding the second hypothesis, the predicted negative correlation between T-Anxiety and moral maturity was found only for boys. Moreover, it is interesting to note that a positive correlation was found for female subjects in a pilot study (there were no male subjects). These results may be interpreted in light of Gilligan's (1982) work on sex differences in moral judgment and her criticism of Kohlberg for not taking gender specificity into account. Gilligan asserted that mature moral judgment for men entails abstract notions of universal moral principles of justice, whereas for women higher stages of maturity may link morality to care and responsibility. This might explain why mature women are higher in T-Anxiety, whereas the opposite pattern appears to hold for men.

Anxiety, Mastectomy, and Hysterectomy

Saba (1982) investigated women's reactions to the threat of mastectomy and hysterectomy. A review of studies of the psychological effects of these surgical procedures have indicated that anxiety is a major reaction to the anticipation of mastectomy and hysterectomy. Spielberger's state–trait anxiety theory provides a meaningful theoretical framework for this research because it distinguishes between anxiety as a situational reaction to surgery and as a personality disposition that may predict postsurgery reactions of depression. Within the framework of this theory, the following hypothesis were tested: (a) An experimental condition evocative of the threat of mastectomy will lead to higher S-Anxiety than a neutral situation; (b) an experimental situation evocative of the threat of hysterectomy will lead to higher S-Anxiety than a neutral situation; and (c) an experimental condition evocative of mastectomy will be more threatening and lead to higher S-Anxiety than the threat of hysterectomy.

The rationale for these hypotheses is that although both kinds of surgery are mutilating and threatening to feminine identity and self-esteem, mastectomy should lead to higher anxiety because the external physical damage it causes is more evident, whereas hysterectomy does not harm the outward appearance of the body in such a radical way. Moreover, having children does not seem to be as important a value nowadays, because women can experience considerable satisfaction and self-fulfillment from work achievement.

The subjects in this study were 165 randomly selected female students from a university in Rio de Janeiro. The design included two fictitious experimental situations, using stories of young women who were told by their physicians that they would have to undergo either a mastectomy or a hysterectomy. These stories were coupled with slides depicting the bodies of women before and after the two kinds of surgery. The subjects were asked to imagine themselves in the place of the woman in the story, and to respond to the STAI as they thought that women would respond. In the control condition, the subjects were asked to respond to the STAI in a neutral condition.

The resulting data were evaluated by means of ANOVA. All three hypotheses were confirmed. Implications for dealing with hysterectomy and mastectomy patients were discussed, especially the critical importance of the medical doctors' sensitivity to the psychological aspects of these kinds of surgery. Physicians must be prepared to deal with the anxieties of hysterectomy and mastectomy patients in regard to their feminine identity.

Anxiety, Self-Concept, and Social Comparisons

In his theory of social comparison, Festinger (1954) hypothesized that individuals tend to compare their opinions and abilities with those of other people. The more secure individuals are in regard to their self-concept, the more likely they are to seek information to support the accuracy of their beliefs or actions. In other words, individuals who are more secure are more likely to engage in a social-comparison process. Moreover, when placed in situations that involve the possibility of social comparison, individuals with high self-esteem appear to be less debilitated by this prospect and more likely to engage in a social comparison process. In contrast, in situations involving social comparison, persons with low self-esteem are likely to find such settings more noxious and anxiety arousing.

Biaggio, Crano, and Crano (1984) investigated relations between self-concept and state–trait anxiety under different levels of social comparison pressure. The main hypothesis of this study was that persons with poor self-concepts will respond to social comparison with higher levels of S-Anxiety than individuals with positive self-concept. Similarly, Spielberger, Gorsuch, and Lushene (1970) have observed that the level of T-Anxiety of individuals with negative self-concepts is higher than that of individuals with positive self-concepts.

The subjects were 31 students (14 boys and 17 girls) from a seventh-grade school in Porto Alegre. Scores on the Janis and Field (1959) self-concept scale (Eagly's, 1967 revision, adapted to Portuguese by Crano & Crano, 1985) were available from a recent study. In the social comparison experimental condition, the subjects were told that they would take a creativity test and that their scores would be compared with those of students from several countries. Subjects in the control group were told that the creativity test was being administered for purposes of checking its validity for Brazilian students. Following the experimental manipulation, the Portuguese STAI was administered to both groups.

The mean S-Anxiety score of the low self-concept subjects in the social comparison condition ($M = 35.17$) was significantly higher than that of high self-concept subjects in the same experimental condition ($M = 28.44$, $t = 2.15$, $p < .05$), whereas there were no differences in the control group in S-Anxiety as a function of self-concept. The correlation between S-Anxiety and self-concept was .72 ($p < .01$) in the social comparison condition, but only .38 (ns) in the control group. For all subjects combined, the mean T-Anxiety score of low self-concept subjects (M = 40.50) was significantly higher (t = 8.85, p < .01) than that for high self-concept subjects (M = 37.35). The correlation between T-Anxiety and self-concept was −.59 (p < .01) for all subjects combined.

The results were discussed in terms of their relevance for Festinger's social comparison theory, Spielberger's trait–state anxiety theory, and the self-concept construct. Implications for education in terms of evaluation practices were also discussed, as it was demonstrated that low self-concept subjects became more anxious under conditions of social comparison. Thus, grading on the curve and other comparative techniques may be detrimental to their learning experience.

SUMMARY

This chapter described the construction and validation of the adult and children's forms of the Portuguese adaptations of the State–Trait Anxiety Inventory (STAI and STAIC, respectively). The psychometric properties of these scales are described in detail in the manuals that are available from the test publisher in Rio de Janeiro (Centro Editor de Psicologia Aplicada [CEPA]). Overviews of investigations in which the Portuguese STAI and STAIC were used to test hypotheses of theoretical interest regarding the relation between state and trait anxiety and locus of control, moral judgment, self-concept, and social comparison were presented. The findings in a study of women's reactions to the threat of mastectomy and hysterectomy were also described.

REFERENCES

Archer, R. P. (1979). Relationships between locus of control, trait-anxiety, and state-anxiety: An interactional perspective. *Journal of Personality, 47,* 305–316.

Biaggio, A. (1967). *Relationships among behavioral, cognitive, and affective aspects of children's conscience.* Unpublished doctoral dissertation, University of Wisconsin.

Biaggio, A. (1980). Desenvolvimento da forma infantil em portugues do Inventario de Ansiedade Traco-Estado de Spielberger [Development of the Portuguese form of Spielberger's STAIC]. *Arquivos Brasileiros de Psicologia, 32,* 106–118.

Biaggio, A. (1983). *Manual Para a Forma Experimental Infantil em Portugues [Portuguese STAIC].* Rio de Janeiro, Brazil: CEPA.

Biaggio, A. (1985). Relationships between state-trait anxiety and locus of control: Experimental studies with adults and children. *International Journal of Behavioral Development, 8,* 153–166.

Biaggio, A. (1990). Relationships between maturity of moral judgment and state-trait anxiety. In Z. Kulscar, C. D. Spielberger, & I. G. Sarason (Eds.), *Stress and anxiety* (Vol. 13, in press). Washington, DC: Hemisphere.

Biaggio, A., Crano, W. E., & Crano, S. L. (1984). Relationships between self-concept and state-trait anxiety under different conditions of social comparison. In C. D. Spielberger and R. Diaz-Guerrero (Eds.), *Cross-cultural anxiety* (Vol. 3, pp. 11–20). Washington, DC: Hemisphere/McGraw-Hill.

Biaggio, A., & Natalicio, L. (1979). *Manual Inventário de Ansiedade: Traco-Estado* [Portuguese STAI]. Rio de Janeiro, Brazil: CEPA.

Biaggio, A., & Natalicio, L., & Spielberger, C. D. (1976). The development and validation of an experimental Portuguese form of the State–Trait Anxiety Inventory. In C. D. Spielberger & R. Diaz-Guerrero (Eds.), *Cross-cultural anxiety* (Vol. 1, pp. 29–40). Washington, DC: Hemisphere.

Blatt, M., & Kohlberg, L. (1975). The effects of classroom moral discussion upon children's level of moral judgment. *Journal of Moral Education, 4,* 129–161.

Bzuneck, J. A. (1979). *Julgamento moral de adolescentes dilinquentes e nao-dilinguentes em relacao com ausencia paterna.* Unpublished doctoral dissertation, Universidade de Sao Paulo, Brazil.

Crano, S. L., & Crano, S. E. (1985). Development of a Portuguese language measure of self-concept. *Interamerican Journal of Psychology,* 122–130.

Cronbach L. J. (1951). Coefficient alpha and the internal structure of tests. *Psychometrika, 16,* 297–335.

Eagly, A. H. (1967). Involvement as a determinant of response to favorable and unfavorable information [Monograph]. *Journal of Personality and Social Psychology, 7,* 1–15.

Feres, N. A. L. (1982). *Locus de controle e comparacao social na atribuicao de causalidade por criangas* [Locus of control and social comparison in attribution of causality by children]. Unpublished doctoral dissertation, Fundacao Getulio Vargas, Rio de Janeiro, Brazil.

Festinger, L. (1954). A theory of social comparison processes. *Human Relations, 7,* 117–140.

Gilligan, C. (1982). *In a different voice.* Cambridge, MA: Harvard University Press.

Janis, I. L., & Field, P. B. (1959). The Janis-Field feelings of inadequacy scale. In I. Janis & C. I. Hovland (Eds.), *Personality and persuasibility.* New Haven, CT: Yale University Press.

Jolley, M. T., & Spielberger, C. D. (1973). The effects of locus of control and anxiety on verbal conditioning. *Journal of Personality, 41,* 443–456.

Kacelnik, E., Oliveira, E. S., & Farias, M. E. (1975). *Relationships between cognitive dissonance and anxiety.* Unpublished senior research paper, Pontificia Universidade Catolica do Rio de Janeiro, Brazil.

Kohlberg, L. (1963). The development of children's orientation toward a moral order: I. Sequence in the development of moral thought. *Vita Humana, 6,* 11–33.

Kohlberg, L. (1981). *Essays on moral development* (Vol. 1). San Francisco: Harper & Row.

Lefcourt, H. M. (1976). *Locus of control: Current trends in theory and research.* Hillsdale, NJ: Erlbaum.

Milgram, N. A. (1971). Locus of control in Negro and White children at four age levels. *Psychological Reports, 29,* 450–465.

Milgram, N. A., & Milgram, R. M. (1975). Dimensions of locus of control in children. *Psychological Reports, 37,* 532–538.

Rest, J. (1976). New approaches in the assessment of moral judgment. In T. Lickona (Eds.), *Moral development and behavior: Theory, research, and social issues.* New York: Holt, Rinehart & Winston.

Rotter, J. B. (1966). Generalized expectancies for internal versus external control of reinforcement. *Psychological Monographs, 80* (1. Serial No. 609).

Rotter, J. B. (1975). Some problems and misconceptions related to the construct of internal versus external reinforcement. *Journal of Consulting and Clinical Psychology, 43,* 56–67.

Saba, A. M. F. (1982). *Reacoes de ansiedade de mulheres perante a mastectomia e a histerectomia.* Unpublished master's thesis, Universidade Federal do Rio de Janeiro, Brazil.

Soares, C. M. F. B. (1977). *Relacionamento entre locus de controle e dependencia-independencia de campo em licieneors da Rucuidade de Educacao de UFRJ.* Unpublished master's thesis, Universidade Federal do Rio de Janeiro, Brazil.

Spielberger, C. D. (1966). Theory and research on anxiety. In C. D. Spielberger (Ed.), *Anxiety and behavior* (pp. 3–20). New York: Academic Press.

Spielberger, C. D. (1972). Anxiety as an emotional state. In C. D. Spielberger (Ed.), *Anxiety: Current trends in theory and research* (Vol. 1, pp. 23–29). New York: Academic Press.

Spielberger, C. D. (1973). *State-Trait Anxiety Inventory for Children: A preliminary manual.* Palo Alto, CA: Consulting Psychologists Press.

Spielberger, C. D., Auerbach, S. M., Wadsworth, A. P., Dunn, T. M., & Taulbee, E. S. (1973). Emotional reactions to surgery. *Journal of Consulting and Clinical Psychology, 40,* 33–38.

Spielberger, C. D., Gorsuch, R. L., & Lushene, R. E. (1970). *Manual for the State-Trait Anxiety Inventory.* Palo Alto, CA: Consulting Psychologists Press.

Steitz, J. A. (1982). Locus of control as a life-span developmental process: Revision of the construct. *International Journal of Behavioral Development, 5,* 299–316.

Taruma, H., Fernandez, E., & Paschoal, C. R. (1975). *STAI scores of surgical patients: A validation study.* Unpublished senior research paper, Pontificia Universidade Católica do Rio de Janeiro, Brazil.

Turiel, E. (1969). Developmental processes in the child's moral thinking. In P. Mussen, J. Langer, & M. Covington (Eds.), *New directions in developmental psychology.* New York: Holt, Rinehart & Winston.

14

Psychometric Properties and Research with the Norwegian State–Trait Anxiety Inventory

Kjell Haseth
University of Oslo, Norway

Knut A. Hagtvet
University of Bergen, Norway

Charles D. Spielberger
University of South Florida, USA

Over the past 20 years, interest among Norwegian psychologists and psychiatrists in stress, anxiety, and related emotional phenomena has greatly increased. Significant progress has also been made in the assessment and treatment of symptoms of stress and anxiety. Moreover, health personnel working in stress-management programs in Norway have become more sophisticated in evaluating the anxiety of their patients and have used a variety of psychological measures to augment and refine their clinical judgments.

The procedures used in the mid-1970s for the assessment of anxiety included behavior rating scales, projective techniques such as the Rorschach and the Thematic Apperception Test, and the Minnesota Multiphasic Personality Inventory, which was used primarily by military psychologists (Hansen, 1985). The limitations in the available measures stimulated Kjell Haseth to develop a Norwegian adaptation of the State–Trait Anxiety Inventory (STAI; Spielberger, Gorsuch, & Lushene, 1970) in order to augment clinical observations and self-ratings of anxiety in phobic patients.

The first step in constructing a Norwegian form of the STAI (the STAI-N) was to translate and adapt the items so that they corresponded conceptually, as closely as possible, with the American originals. The clarity of the translations was ascertained by reviewing alternative formulations of each item with colleagues who were trained as psychologists in the United States. The equivalence of the Norwegian adaptation of the STAI with the American original was demonstrated by administering the STAI and the STAI-N to bilingual students (Haseth, 1978). The clinical applicability of the STAI-N has been demonstrated in measuring the anxiety of phobic patients.

RESEARCH WITH EARLY ADAPTATIONS
OF THE NORWEGIAN STAI

The STAI-N was first used in the field of catastrophy psychiatry. Lars Weisæth (1984) and his colleagues individually administered the STAI-N State Anxiety (S-Anxiety) Scale to 246 victims of an explosion in a large paint factory. Elevated STAI-N S-Anxiety scores predicted whether a particular victim would develop a posttraumatic stress disorder (PTSD). In repeated evaluations of persons receiving treatment for PTSD, state anxiety, as measured by the STAI-N S-Anxiety Scale, was found to correspond closely to overall clinical judgments (Weisæth, 1984). The STAI-N is now routinely used in Norway to assess anxiety in a variety of clinical settings by a team of catastrophy psychiatry personnel headed by Weisæth.

A research group at the University of Bergen used the STAI-N in an extensive series of job stress and adjustment studies (Ursin, 1980; Ursin, Baade, & Levine, 1978). Short- and long-term effects of job stress on autonomic arousal, anxiety, self-reported stress symptoms, hormonal changes, defensive and coping strategies, and the immune system have been investigated. Findings in these studies demonstrated that variations in activation were related to several psychological parameters, including S-Anxiety. The original STAI-N has also been used to assess the anxiety of pregnant women (Bjorseth & Warncke, 1985) and in studies of various occupational groups, such as nurses (Endresen, 1984), divers (Arnestad & Aanestad, 1985; Vaernes, 1982), lifeboat crews (Relling, 1983), firefighters (Hilldal & Solbue, 1986), and so forth.

A slightly modified version of the Norwegian STAI (Form X), developed by Hagtvet (1984b), was used in a longitudinal study of pregnancy (Valand, 1986). As expected, S-Anxiety scores reflected an increase in the intensity of S-Anxiety during pregnancy and labor. On the other hand, trait anxiety (T-Anxiety) was remarkably stable. When these data were evaluated by means of covariance structural modeling (Hagtvet, 1986; Valand & Hagtvet, 1987), the findings supported Spielberger's (1966, 1972) trait–state anxiety theory. The T-Anxiety Scale appeared to measure stable individual differences during pregnancy, whereas scores on the S-Anxiety seemed to assess both change and stability.

The Hagtvet (1984b) version of the STAI (Form X) has also been used in a number of studies of test anxiety in university students, and in eighth- and ninth-grade pupils in the Norwegian school system. In a validation study of the Norwegian adaptation of Spielberger's (1980) Test Anxiety Inventory, Hagtvet (1984a) found that the STAI-N S-Anxiety Scale was more strongly and consistently related to emotionality than to worry in three different groups of students (Hagtvet, 1983, 1984a, 1984c, 1985, 1988a).

Reiersen and Svebak (1987) found that T-Anxiety was unrelated to somatic complaints (e.g., palpitations, tingling) in university students who were given a hyperventilation provocation test, but high T-Anxiety subjects reported more emotional complaints. In another experiment with students, Nysveen (1986) investigated the relation between S-Anxiety scores and the labeling of physiological responses (heart rate and skin conductance level) during an evaluative test situation. Although the physiological reactions were not related to state anxiety in this study, Vassend (1987) demonstrated that examination stress produced an increase in state anxiety.

The relation between hypnotizability, imaginative involvement (absorption), and anxiety responses was examined by Vassend and Nysveen (1987), who reported a small positive correlation ($r = .26$) between S-Anxiety and self-ratings of global hypnotic depth. However, S-Anxiety was not related to hypnotic susceptibility and capacity for imaginative involvement. The STAI has also been used in Norway in several studies of exercise and mental health. Dagmund Svensen translated the STAI into *nynorsk*—a form of the Norwegian language used by approximately 18% of the population (Vaa, 1982).

The results of an exploratory factor analysis of the Form X version of the STAI indicated that simple structure was approximated when three or four factors were extracted (Hagtvet, 1988b). These solutions also provided psychologically meaningful interpretations. The four-factor solution yielded the factors T-Anxiety Present, T-Anxiety Absent, S-Anxiety Present, and S-Anxiety Absent. However, simple structure was best in the three-factor solution, which yielded T-Anxiety, S-Anxiety Present, and S-Anxiety Absent factors. The three-factor solution was also more strongly supported in a second-order confirmatory factor solution.

In a follow-up study, the STAI was administered to a random sample of 441 university students in a relatively relaxed situation, that is, the students were registering for the spring term. Four sum scores were formed to measure the four factors identified by Hagtvet (1988b): S-Anxiety Present, S-Anxiety Absent, T-Anxiety Present, and T-Anxiety Absent (Hagtvet, Reiersen, & Svebak, 1987). Consistent with Spielberger's item-intensity specificity hypothesis (Spielberger et al., 1970), an interaction effect was found for the two anxiety-absent measures that reflected an interesting gender difference. Women scored higher than men, but only within married student couples.

Psychologists and psychiatrists in Norway are presently using the STAI extensively, and interest in the inventory is growing. Three somewhat different versions of the scale are in current use. Although the instructions, the scale format, and most of the items are similar in the three versions, the response categories are different. The existence of three different Norwegian versions of the STAI leads to confusion in interpreting experimental findings. Moreover, all three versions were based on the original English version, which has been extensively revised (Spielberger, 1983). Therefore, the time seemed right to develop a definitive Norwegian adaptation of the STAI.

PROCEDURE FOR ADAPTING
THE REVISED STAI (FORM Y) IN NORWEGIAN

On the basis of conceptual clarification gained from a decade of research with the STAI (Form X), 12 of the 40 Form X items were replaced in constructing the revised STAI (Form Y), the latest revised form of the inventory (Spielberger, 1980). Some of the replaced items had been found to be ambiguous, and several with content more closely related to depression than to anxiety (e.g., "I feel blue" and "I feel like crying") were replaced. The revised STAI (Form Y) has a better balance in the T-Anxiety Scale of anxiety-absent and anxiety-present items. The factor structure and psychometric properties of the S-Anxiety and T-Anxiety scales were also improved.

In translating and adapting the STAI (Form Y) into Norwegian, the first step was to select the best items from the earlier Norwegian versions and to translate the new STAI (Form Y) items into Norwegian. The format of the Norwegian adaptation closely resembles the English STAI test form. Essentially the same instructions were used as in the earlier versions of the Norwegian STAI (Form X) (Haseth, 1978). The 4-point frequency rating scale for the revised Norwegian T-Anxiety Scale was the same as in the earlier Norwegian form; the S-Anxiety Scale of the STAI-N (Form Y) was simplified and improved, following suggestions made by Weisæth (1984), because of the difficulty experienced with highly anxious individuals. The categories for the 4-point intensity scale were (a) *aldeles ikke* (not at all), (b) *litt* (somewhat), (c) *noksa mye* (moderately so), and (d) *svaert mye* (very much so).

The second step in constructing the Norwegian STAI (Form Y) was to develop an item pool. Items from the Norwegian STAI (Form X) that had been previously shown to have good psychometric properties were included without alteration (Hagtvet, 1984a, 1988b); alternative translations were included for those Norwegian STAI (Form X) items that previous research had shown to be ambiguous. Several translations were also written for each new STAI (Form Y) item (Spielberger, 1983). Thus, the item pool for the STAI-N (Form Y) consisted of a larger number of items than would be required in the final version.

The preliminary Norwegian scale was administered to a large group of medical and psychology students at the University of Oslo during a regular class period and to recruits at the Oslo Police Academy. Following the traditional procedure recommended by Spielberger (1983, p. 4), the S-Anxiety Scale was administered before the T-Anxiety Scale. The students were first asked to respond to the S-Anxiety Scale by reporting their feelings at the moment (a standard instruction). They were then asked to respond to the S-Anxiety Scale while they imagined themselves to be in a situation just before an important exam or job interview. Finally, they were given the T-Anxiety Scale with standard instructions. These procedures were essentially the same as those used by Spielberger et al. (1970). Thus, the internal consistency reliability for responses to the English and Norwegian forms of the test given under relaxed and vicarious stressful test-taking conditions could be compared for Norwegian and American students.

PSYCHOMETRIC PROPERTIES
OF THE NORWEGIAN STAI

In gathering normative data for the Norwegian STAI (Form Y), the preliminary version of the test was administered during an ordinary lecture to large groups of psychology and medical students, aged 19–24 years (200 women and 97 men). The testing session was considered nonstressful as the next exam was at least 2 months away and the students were told that only group data would be reported. The preliminary STAI-N (Form Y) was also administered to 241 first-year recruits at a police academy (65 women and 176 men), aged 19–24 years, who were tested in regular classrooms in groups of 20–30. This testing situation was considered more stressful than the one for college students because a major exam was scheduled in 2 weeks and the recruits were less accustomed to taking psychological tests. To reduce some of the inherent stress, the recruits were told that their responses to the test would be anonymous and that only group results would be reported.

The means, standard deviations, and alpha coefficients for the two groups are presented in Table 1. It can be seen that the T-Anxiety scores were higher than the S-Anxiety scores for the university students and the female police recruits. Similar findings were reported by Spielberger (1983), which were interpreted as evidence that the test situation was nonstressful. For the male recruits, the difference between the T-Anxiety and the S-Anxiety scores was essentially zero, suggesting that these subjects were somewhat more aroused and on guard during the test administration than were the other groups.

It may also be noted in Table 1 that the T-Anxiety scores of the women were generally higher than those of the comparable group of men. These differences were most pronounced for the police recruits ($t = 3.49$, $p < .001$), but were also significant for the college students ($t = 2.52$, $p < .01$). In addition, women obtained higher S-Anxiety scores than men, but these gender differences were not statistically significant. These findings are similar to the results reported for college students and military recruits by other researchers (Spielberger, 1983; van der Ploeg, 1985).

RELIABILITY AND VALIDITY OF THE NORWEGIAN STAI (FORM Y)

The reliability of the STAI has been evaluated by investigating test–retest scores or the scales' internal consistency. According to Spielberger (1972, 1985), state anxiety would be expected to fluctuate over time as a function of situational stress. Consequently, S-Anxiety scores on any two occasions might reflect differences in perceived situational stress rather than indicating the unreliability of the test. In contrast, because trait-anxiety measures are expected to reflect relatively stable individual differences in anxiety proneness, high test–retest stability would be expected for the STAI T-Anxiety Scale, and higher test–retest stability has been observed for the STAI T-Anxiety Scale than for the S-Anxiety Scale in several empirical investigations (e.g., Spielberger, 1983; van der Ploeg, 1985).

Information about the test–retest reliability of the Norwegian STAI (Form Y) is lacking, but the Cronbach's alpha coefficients reported in Tables 1 and 2 provide a

Table 1 Means, Standard Deviations, and Cronbach's Alpha Reliabilities on the Norwegian STAI (Form Y) for College Students and Police Academy Recruits

Scale	College students		Police academy recruits	
	Men	Women	Men	Women
State anxiety				
N	97	200	176	65
M	34.25	35.95	29.23	30.76
SD	8.33	10.27	6.00	6.35
Alpha	.90	.93	.87	.88
Trait anxiety				
N	97	200	176	65
M	36.08	39.17	29.64	32.98
SD	9.50	10.12	6.01	7.99
Alpha	.93	.93	.84	.93

Table 2 Item-Remainder Correlations for the State–Trait Anxiety Inventory Scale for College Students and Recruits at the Police Academy

Item number	College students		Police recruits		Item number	College students		Police recruits	
	Men	Women	Men	Women		Men	Women	Men	Women
	State Anxiety Scale					Trait Anxiety Scale			
1	55	70	49	75	21	70	76	59	67
2	70	69	58	69	22	68	59	42	53
3	60	65	44	55	23	72	68	54	65
4	35	69	41	32	24	40	53	34	65
5	74	69	57	50	25	61	58	32	66
6	35	48	43	37	26	46	49	36	59
7	32	60	57	40	27	70	61	50	69
8	69	75	54	61	28	66	63	42	64
9	46	57	35	40	29	43	60	29	51
10	53	67	48	48	30	63	67	61	61
11	56	63	54	54	31	56	56	34	45
12	57	60	43	53	32	68	65	27	68
13	34	64	25	46	33	63	73	52	68
14	61	39	43	41	34	55	40	32	42
15	62	69	57	54	35	57	58	38	61
16	62	71	55	37	36	77	74	71	68
17	39	58	40	47	37	34	51	32	63
18	57	61	36	20	38	59	53	33	63
19	47	68	55	44	39	73	63	47	51
20	67	71	46	70	40	58	66	38	64
Mdn	57	65	54	53	*Mdn*	63	61	42	64
Alpha	90	93	87	88	Alpha	93	93	84	93

Note. Item numbers refer to Spielberger's official STAI (Form Y format). Decimal points have been omitted.

measure of the internal consistency and reliability of these scales. The reliabilities varied between .84 and .93, indicating that the adapted scales show the same high level of internal consistency as the original English form and other adaptations around the world. The lowest alpha reliability was observed for male police recruits (.87 for the S-Anxiety Scale and .84 for the T-Anxiety scale), which was consistent with the lower means and smaller standard deviations for this group.

Item-remainder correlations for the individual items in the final version of the Norwegian STAI (Form Y) are reported in Table 2. With few exceptions, each S-Anxiety and the T-Anxiety item correlated highly with the respective subscale score. For the college students, these correlations were all above .30, and the median item-remainder correlations were between .57 and .65. Although several correlations for the police academy groups were below .30, the median for these groups was .54. The alpha of .84 for male recruits may reflect their lower educational level.

The adaptation of the Norwegian STAI (Form Y) was begun only 2 years ago, and only limited data are available for evaluating the scales' validity. However, previous research with the Norwegian STAI (Form X) has demonstrated good concurrent and content validity (Hagtvet, 1984a, 1988b; Heggestad & Ronold, 1983; Relling, 1983). Because 70% of the Norwegian STAI (Form Y) items were taken from the STAI-N (Form X) with only minimal alteration, the improvement in the psychometric properties of Form Y should enhance the validity of this form.

Evidence of the construct validity of the Norwegian STAI (Form Y) was provided for a subgroup of college students who completed the scale with standard instructions, and who also responded to the scale while imagining themselves shortly before an important examination or job interview. The same procedure was followed by Spielberger et al. (1970), using college students as subjects. As can be seen in Table 3, the S-Anxiety scores of both American and Norwegian students were significantly higher under the imagined stressful condition than in the normal test-taking condition. Table 4 shows that the mean scores for the stressful condition were higher than those in the neutral condition for all of the items in the American study, and were significantly higher for all but one of the Norwegian STAI (Form Y) items. The degree to which each item reflected differences in S-Anxiety on the two test occasions is indicated by the size of the reported *t* values for the Norwegian students.

Spielberger et al. (1970) referred to differences in the sensitivity of specific items to different kinds and degrees of stress as *item intensity specificity*. He later suggested (Spielberger, 1985) that anxiety-absent items ("I feel at ease," "I am relaxed") were more sensitive at lower levels of stress, whereas anxiety-present items ("I feel upset," "I feel nervous") were more sensitive at higher stress levels ($p < .15$). By examining differences in item-remainder correlations obtained under neutral and stressful conditions, Spielberger et al. (1970) identified some items as more sensitive under neutral conditions as compared with stressful conditions, and vice versa. In our study of Norwegian students, we were also able to identify certain items as having differential sensitivity in the two testing conditions.

As can be seen in Table 5, anxiety-absent items 5 and 16, "I feel at ease (*Jeg foler meg vel*)" and "I feel content (*Jeg er fornoyd*)," are more sensitive to variations in S-Anxiety at the lower intensity range as determined by the magnitude of the correlations of these items with the scale as a whole on the measurement occasions. Anxiety-present items 6 and 9, "I feel upset (*Jeg foler meg oppskaket*)" and "*I feel frightened* (Jeg foler meg skremt)," were more sensitive at the higher portions of the intensity range (Table 5). Although some items with differential sensitivity were identified, most of the items were equally sensitive in both the normal and the stressful condition.

In adapting the STAI for another language or culture, one might raise the ques-

Table 3 Mean State Anxiety Scores (Sum Scores) for American and Norwegian College Students

Students' nationality and gender	*n*	Norm	Exam	CR	r_{pb}
American					
Male	332	40.02	54.99	24.14	.60
Female	645	39.36	60.51	42.13	.73
Norwegian					
Male	56	34.26	56.25	$p < .001$	
Female	116	35.97	61.48	$p < .001$	

Note. Data on American students reported by Spielberger et al. (1970).

Table 4 Mean Scores on State Anxiety Items under Normal and Anxiety Provoked Test Administration in American and Norwegian College Students

Item number	Men					Women				
	American students		Norwegian students			American students		Norwegian students		
	Norm	Exam	Norm	Exam	*t*	Norm	Exam	Norm	Exam	*t*
				Anxiety-absent items						
1	1.90	3.11	1.94	3.50	12.58	1.85	3.42	1.94	3.53	15.89
2	2.17	2.95	1.92	3.21	10.94	2.16	3.20	1.98	3.41	15.52
5	2.07	3.11	2.07	3.39	12.92	2.04	3.39	2.00	3.48	14.96
8*	2.86	2.92	2.14	3.32	12.31	2.93	3.07	2.12	3.52	13.17
10	2.44	3.01	2.44	3.54	8.68	2.20	3.14	2.36	3.77	15.83
11	2.19	2.73	1.98	2.63	5.45	2.42	3.10	2.22	3.03	9.74
15	2.27	3.07	2.09	3.48	10.21	2.27	3.37	2.23	3.68	17.48
16	2.38	3.10	2.25	3.18	8.23	2.35	3.37	2.06	3.49	15.10
19*	2.80	3.56	2.03	2.86	6.86	2.63	3.74	2.19	3.12	10.47
20	2.36	3.13	1.85	3.30	13.38	2.07	3.25	1.90	3.42	16.93
				Anxiety-present items						
3	1.63	2.97	1.59	3.23	12.54	1.65	3.29	1.77	3.43	18.54
4*	1.35	2.12	1.48	3.19	15.15	1.29	2.31	1.61	3.25	16.29
6	1.30	2.08	1.23	2.25	7.62	1.31	2.48	1.23	2.63	13.19
7	1.95	2.67	1.23	1.84	5.83	1.84	2.87	1.51	2.38	7.28
9*	2.46	2.71	1.07	2.05	7.95	2.48	3.13	1.19	2.48	12.81
12	1.68	2.76	1.34	2.79	11.61	1.68	3.12	1.38	3.09	17.17
13	1.41	2.28	1.10	2.29	9.23	1.39	2.68	1.15	2.80	17.66
14*	1.42	1.97	1.71	2.10	3.39	1.37	2.25	1.71	2.03	3.56
17	2.02	2.80	1.48	2.34	7.44	2.13	3.15	1.78	2.89	11.37
18*	1.29	1.93	1.54	1.76	1.94	1.23	2.19	1.52	2.03	5.52

Note. For Norwegian students, the results of the *t* tests are reported for every item. Norwegian sample—116 women, 54 men (based on Form Y); American sample—88 women, 109 men (based on Form X; Spielberger et al., 1970).

*Items replaced in Form Y.

tion as to how much attention should be paid to the item intensity specificity phenomenon. The Norwegian data seem to indicate that by sticking closely to the American originals when translating items, the items that are chosen are likely to cover the entire range of intensity. In selecting S-Anxiety items for special purposes (e.g., testing highly anxious individuals), knowledge about differential item sensitivity could be used in making up an instrument that was especially sensitive at the desired intensity range. In a study of Norwegians characterized by abnormally high anxiety levels, Weisæth (1984) found that their reactions to one particular anxiety-present item ("I am jittery [*Jeg er skvetten*"]) was most sensitive in reflecting both the initial anxiety level and later recovery.

FACTOR STRUCTURE OF THE NORWEGIAN STAI

Numerous studies have investigated the factor structure of the STAI (Spielberger, 1983). In most studies in which all 40 items were factored simultaneously, two separate state- and trait-anxiety dimensions were identified. Because there was some disagreement as to the factor structure of the STAI (Form X; Endler & Edwards, 1985), Spielberger revised the scales and performed several factor studies to clarify the structure of the STAI (Form Y; Spielberger, Vagg, Barker, Donham, & Westberry, 1980; Vagg, Spielberger, & O'Hearn, 1980). In these studies, four factors could be readily identified; S-Anxiety Absent, S-Anxiety Present, T-Anxiety Absent, and T-Anxiety Present. In Norway, two factor studies of the STAI (Form X) have been reported. Vaa (1982) used children as subjects and observed a clear state–trait distinction with fairly good three- and four-factor solutions. Similar findings have been reported by Hagtvet (1988b).

In the present study, only the female sample met the requirement of a sufficient number of cases (n = 200) to allow a meaningful exploratory factor analysis (Gorsuch, 1974). Factors were extracted by means of principal-axis method, using the SPSS package (Nie, Hull, Jenkins, Steinbrenner, & Bent, 1975), with rotation by the normalized varimax procedure. Although the scree test criterion suggested that three factors could be extracted, results from the two-, three-, and four-factor solutions were inspected with respect to simple structure and psychological meaningfulness.

The two-factor solution yielded a clear state–trait factor structure, as can be seen in Table 6. The exception seems to be Item 11, "I feel self-confident (*Jeg er sikker på meg selv*)," which had salient loadings not only on the expected state factor but also on the trait factor. Several double loadings were also observed in the three- and four-factor solutions, which are also reported in Table 6. One possible explanation for these double loadings may be that the Norwegian equivalent of the English "I am," instead of "I feel," was used. Perhaps the "I am" formulation led subjects to confound the intensity of the feeling with frequency of occurrence.

As can be noted in Table 6, the three-factor solution seemed to produce better simple structure than the four-factor solution. With the exeption of Item 11, the trait factor came out satisfactorily. The other two factors were defined by state-absent and state-present items, respectively. Each absent and present item had its highest loadings on the expected factor, but a few items also had salient but smaller loadings on the other factor.

In the four-factor solution, the following factors were identified: T-Anxiety, S-Anxiety Absent, S-Anxiety Present, and what we have termed a *Worry-Oriented*

Table 5   Item-Remainder Correlations for Two Anxiety Absent Items (5 and 16) and two Anxiety Present Items (6 and 9) under Normal and Stress Conditions (116 Female and 56 Male College Students)

Item number	Normal		Stress	
	Men	Women	Men	Women
5	69	74	41	65
16	71	62	47	44
6	35	48	49	71
9	45	57	61	69

Table 6 Varimax-Rotated Factor Structure of the Norwegian State–Trait Anxiety Inventory (Form Y) for 200 Female College Students

Item number	Two-factor solution		Three-factor solution			Four-factor solution			
	1	2	1	2	3	1	2	3	4
1	70			58	45		55	46	
2	63			58			54		
3	67				68			61	
4	61				57	51			
5	66			70		72			
6	51				53			54	
7	55				60			58	
8	71			71		77			
9	57				58			62	
10	64			64		65			
11	48	52	47			48	43		
12	62				63			72	
13	52				53			63	
14	(30)				(31)				(37)
15	69			57	43	56	41		
16	66			71		73			
17	53				55				50
18	59				54			47	
19	63			52	40	52			
20	65			66		67			
21		76	72		41	79			
22		47	46		42	(38)			
23		68	64	41	41	69			
24		55	54			51			
25		55	52			48			
26		41	38			(36)			
27		53	49			51			
28		56	56			42			
29		51	52		41			58	
30		65	61			64			
31		53	54			41			43
32		62	61			56			
33		71	67	41		74			
34		(37)	(36)			(30)			
35		56	54			49			
36		74	71			76			
37		52	55						49
38		54	56			46			
39		59	56			60			
40		59	58			44			50
Factor name	S-Anxiety	T-Anxiety	T-Anxiety	S-Anxiety Absent	S-Anxiety Present	T-Anxiety	S-Anxiety Absent	S-Anxiety Present	Worry
Unrotated eigenvalue	14.72	3.22	14.72	3.22	2.14	14.72	3.22	2.15	1.42

Note. Only loadings above .40 are reported. For items with no salient loadings, highest loadings are indicated in parentheses. Decimal points have been omitted. Items 1–20 are state items; Items 20–40 are trait items. S-Anxiety = state anxiety; T-Anxiety = trait anxiety.

factor. This fourth factor consisted of two S-Anxiety-present and four T-Anxiety-present items. All of the items constituting the Worry-Oriented factor describe worries and disturbing thoughts.

SUMMARY AND CONCLUSIONS

In this chapter, we have reported the findings of several studies in which the Norwegian STAI (Form X) was used. We have also reviewed the available Norwegian literature on the STAI and described the development of a Norwegian form of the revised STAI (Form Y). In general, our findings with regard to the psychometric properties of the Norwegian STAI appear to be quite similar to those reported from other countries.

The most noteworthy deviation of the present study from previous research seems to be that the factor structure of the Norwegian STAI differs somewhat from other adaptations. The results from three independent Norwegian studies suggested that a three-factor solution (one trait and two state factors) best fit the Norwegian data. Although these findings invite speculation about national stereotypes in responding to the trait items, we defer further discussion of this possibility until additional factor analyses can be performed on new samples of high-school-age subjects.

REFERENCES

Arnestad, M., & Aanestad, B. (1985) *Undersokelse av arbeidsmiljoet ved et psykiatrisk sykehus-stress, helse og immunglobulin-niva.* [*An inquiry into the working conditions at a psychiatric hospital— stress, health, and level of immunoglobulin*]. Unpublished masters thesis, University of Bergen, Norway.

Bjorseth, I., & Warncke, M. (1985). *Svangerskap og psykologisk stress* [*Pregnancy and psychological stress*]. Unpublished masters thesis, University of Bergen, Norway.

Endler, N. S., & Edwards, J. M. (1985). Evaluation of the state-trait distinction within an interaction model of personality. *The Southern Psychologist, 2,* 63–71.

Endresen, I. M. (1984). *Stress, helse og immunglobulin—niva hos pleiere ved et somatisk sykehus.* [*Stress, health, and immunoglobulin level in nurses at a general hospital*]. Unpublished masters thesis, University of Bergen, Norway.

Gorsuch, R. L. (1974). *Factor analysis.* Philadelphia: Saunders.

Hagtvet, K. A. (1983). A construct validation study of test anxiety: A discriminant validation of fear of failure, worry and emotionality. In H. M. van der Ploeg, R. Schwarzer, and C. D. Spielberger (Eds.), *Advances in test anxiety research* (Vol. 2, pp. 15–34). Lisse, the Netherlands: Swets/ Erlbaum.

Hagtvet, K. A. (1984a). A Norwegian adaptation of the Test Anxiety Inventory: A first tryout. *International Review of Applied Psychology, 33,* 257–265.

Hagtvet, K. A. (1984b). *A slightly modified version of the Norwegian adaptation of the State-Trait Anxiety Inventory (STAI).* Unpublished report, Department of Psychometrics, University of Bergen, Norway.

Hagtvet, K. A. (1984c). Fear of failure, worry and emotionality: Their suggestive causal relationship to mathematical performance and state anxiety. In H. M. van der Ploeg, R. Schwarzer, & C. D. Spielberger (Eds.), *Advances in test anxiety research* (Vol. 3, pp. 201–210). Lisse, the Netherlands: Swets/Erlbaum.

Hagtvet, K. A. (1985). A three dimensional test anxiety construct: Worry and emotionality as mediating factors between negative motivation and test behavior. In J. J. Sanches-Sosa (Ed.), *Health and clinical psychology* (pp. 161–162). Amsterdam: North-Holland.

Hagtvet, K. A. (1986). A longitudinal model with parameters of stability and change. *Psychological Reports, 60,* 161–162.

Hagtvet, K. A. (1988a). Et tredimensjonalt testangstbegrep: Dets relevans for integrering av ulike forskningstradisjoner [A three dimensional test anxiety construct: Its relevance for integrating different research traditions]. In T. Gjesme & O. Boe (Eds.), *Motivasjon og laering* (pp. 209–232). Oslo, Norway: Norwegian University Press.

Hagtvet, K. A. (1988b, July). *Studies related to item-intensity specificity of anxiety scales.* Paper presented at the 9th annual meeting of the Society for Test Anxiety Research, Padova University, Italy.

Hagtvet, K. A., Reiersen, O. A., & Svebak, S. (1987). *Relations among demographic and psychosocial variables in a random sample of university students.* Unpublished report, Department of Psychometrics, University of Bergen, Norway.

Hansen, I. (1985). En oversikt over den norsk normering av the Minnesota Multiphasic Personality Inventory. *Journal of Norwegian Psychological Association, 23,* 44–56.

Haseth, K. (1978). *The State–Trait Anxiety Inventory—norsk oversettelse og forelopig evaluering av sprak og personlighetsdimensjoner.* Unpublished report, Institute of Psychology, University of Oslo, Norway.

Heggestad, G., & Ronold, K. F. (1983). *Nitrogennarkose og yteevne under hyperbare forhold. En undersokelse av sammenhengen mellom personlighetsvariabler og yteevne hos dykkere. [Nitrogen narcosis and performance. An inquiry into the relation between personality variables and performance in divers].* Unpublished thesis, University of Bergen, Norway.

Hilldal, G., & Solbue, E. (1986). *Brannmenn: Arbeidsmiljo og helse.* Unpublished thesis, University of Bergen, Norway.

Nie, N. H., Hull, C. H., Jenkins, J. G., Steinbrennen, K., & Bent, D. H. (1975). *SPSS: Statistical package for the social sciences.* New York: McGraw-Hill.

Nysveen, G. (1986). *Test-angst: En eksperimentell studie av efferkter ved rebenevne fysiologiske reacsjoner i en evalueringssituasjon* [Test anxiety: An experimental study of effects of relabeling physiolgical responses in an evaluative test situation]. Unpublished masters thesis, University of Oslo, Norway.

Reierson, O. A., & Svebak, S. (1987, June). *State and trait anxiety in hyperventilation-related complaints.* Paper presented at the 8th annual meeting of the Society for Test Anxiety Research, Bergen, Norway.

Relling, G. B. (1983). *Psykologiske og fysiologiske reaksjoner for og etter fall i fritt fall-livbat. [Psychological and physiological reactions before and after a free fall emergency drop of a lifeboat].* Unpublished thesis, University of Bergen, Norway.

Spielberger, C. D. (1966). Theory and research on anxiety. In C. D. Spielberger (Ed.), *Anxiety and behavior* (pp. 3–20). New York: Academic Press.

Spielberger, C. D. (1972). Anxiety as an emotional state. In C. D. Spielberger (Ed.), *Anxiety, current trends in theory and research* (pp. 23–49). New York: Academic Press.

Spielberger, C. D. (1980). *Preliminary professional manual for the Test Anxiety Inventory.* Palo Alto, CA: Consulting Psychologists Press.

Spielberger, C. D. (1983). *Manual for the State–Trait Anxiety Inventory* (Rev. ed.). Palo Alto, CA: Consulting Psychologists Press.

Spielberger, C. D. (1985). Assessment of state and trait anxiety: Conceptual and methodological issues. *The Southern Psychologist, 2,* 6–16.

Spielberger, C. D., Gorsuch, R. L., & Lushene, R. D. (1970). *Manual for the State–Trait Anxiety Inventory (STAI).* Palo Alto, CA: Consulting Psychologists Press.

Spielberger, C. D., Vagg, P. R., Barker, L. R., Donham, G. W., & Westberry, L. G. (1980). The factor structure of the State–Trait Anxiety Inventory. In I. G. Sarason & C. D. Spielberger (Eds.), *Stress and anxiety* (Vol. 7, pp. 95–109). Washington, DC: Hemisphere.

Ursin, H. (1980). Personality, activation and somatic health: A new psychosomatic theory. In S. Levine & H. Ursin (Eds.), *Coping and health.* London: Plenum Press.

Ursin, H., Baade, E., & Levine, S. (1978). *Psychobiology of stress: A study of coping men.* New York: Academic Press.

Vaa, T. (1982). *Standardisering og normering av Spielberger's State–Trait Anxiety Inventory (STAI) pa et utvalg norske 4., 6. og 8. Klassinger. [Standardization of Spielberger's State-Trait Anxiety Inventory on a group of elementary school children in Norway].* Unpublished master's thesis, University of Olso, Norway.

Vaernes, R. J. (1982). The Defense Mechanism Test predicts inadequate performance under stress. *Scandinavian Journal of Psychology, 23,* 37–43.

Vagg, P. R., Spielberger, C. D., & O'Hearn, T. P., Jr. (1980). Is the State-Trait Anxiety Inventory multidimensional? *Personality and Individual Differences, 1,* 202–214.

Valand, B. (1986). *Kvinnens emosjonelle applevelse av svangerskap og fodsel* [Women's experience of pregnancy and labor]. Unpublished thesis, University of Oslo, Norway.

Valand, B., & Hagtvet, K. A. (1987). *Measuring stability and change in anxiety: A longitudinal study encompassing pregnancy and labor.* Paper presented at the 8th annual meeting of the International Society for Test Anxiety Research, Bergen, Norway.

Van der Ploeg, H. M. (1985). The development and validation of the Dutch State–Trait Anxiety Inventory. In C. D. Spielberger, I. G. Sarason, & P. B. Defares (Eds.), *Stress and anxiety* (Vol. 9, pp. 129–139). New York: Hemisphere.

Vassend, O. (1987). *Examination stress, personality and self-reported physical symptoms.* Unpublished report, Institute of Psychology, University of Oslo, Norway.

Vassend, O. & Nysveen, G. (1987). Hypnotizability, imaginative involvement, and anxiety. Institute of Psychology, University of Oslo, Unpublished report.

Weisæth, L. (1984). *Stress reactions to an individual disaster.* Unpublished doctoral dissertation, University of Oslo, Norway.

15

The Relationship of Test Anxiety to Intelligence and Academic Performance

Frantisek Man
Pedagogical Faculty, Ceské Budéjovice, Czechoslovakia

Petr Blahus
Charles University, Prague, Czechoslovakia

Charles D. Spielberger
University of South Florida, USA

Previous research in various countries has shown that high test-anxious students perform more poorly than those with low test anxiety (Man & Hosek, 1989; Sipos, Sipos, & Spielberger, 1985; Spielberger, 1962, 1980; van der Ploeg, 1982, 1983, 1984). However, although some researchers have found moderate negative correlations between test anxiety and performance (e.g., Schwarzer, 1975), others have failed to find any relationship (Krohne, 1980). On the basis of a comprehensive review of test anxiety research in West German schools, Bowler stated, "usually less than 10 percent of the criterion variance is explained by test anxiety" (1982, p. 88).

Intelligence is, of course, positively related to academic grades. However, studies of the interactive effects of anxiety and ability on cognitive performance and complex learning have reported different types of interactions (cf. Hagtvet, 1986). Spielberger (1962) and Gjesme (1972), for example, found a negative relation between anxiety and grades for university students in the broad middle range of ability, whereas Spielberger (1962) and Heinrich (1979) reported a positive relationship between anxiety and performance among high-ability university students.

Differences in the effects of test anxiety and ability on academic achievement have also been reported in cross-cultural research. Gjesme (1972) in Norway and Sharma and Rao (1983) in India reported a negative relation between test anxiety and academic performance for high-ability girls, Van der Ploeg (1984) in The Netherlands found a large negative correlation for high-ability boys, and Gaudry and Fitzgerald (1971) in Australia found no relation between aptitude and performance in high-ability high school students. In addition to the cultural differences,

This chapter reports the findings of papers that were presented by F. Man and P. Blahus at the Ninth International Conference of the International Society for Test Anxiety Research in Padua, Italy, July 1988. We wish to express our appreciation to V. Hosek and I. Novackova for their contributions to the studies that are described in this chapter.

these findings are undoubtedly influenced by considerable variation in the measures used to assess test anxiety and ability, and by a variety of selection factors that determined the characteristics of the samples in the various studies. Consequently, we must agree with Hagtvet (1986) that no meaningful theoretical conclusions can as yet be drawn from this research.

Liebert and Morris (1967) were the first to introduce the conceptualization of test anxiety as consisting of two major components: worry and emotionality. The concept of emotionality refers to a homogeneous psychophysiological pattern (Jerusalem, 1985), composed not only of the physiological arousal, but also of the subjective perception of the experience of an internal affective-physiological state (Schwarzer, Jerusalem, & Lange, 1982, p. 68). Worry seems to refer to a more complex phenomenon, which includes cognitive concerns about performance, the consequences of failure, negative self-evaluation of one's ability as compared with others and so forth (Hagtvet, 1986; Heckhausen, 1982; Hodapp, Laux, & Spielberger, 1982; Sarason, 1975; Wine, 1982). Thus, the worry component of test anxiety may represent more than one factor (cf. Jerusalem, 1985).

The worry–emotionality distinction in test anxiety research has focused on *state* test anxiety (cf. Deffenbacher, 1980; Liebert & Morris, 1967; Morris, Davis, & Hutchings, 1981), with little attention devoted to the question of whether this distinction was also viable with regard to test anxiety as a personality trait. Spielberger (1972) conceptualized test anxiety as a situation-specific anxiety trait and developed the Test Anxiety Inventory (TAI; Spielberger, 1980) to measure individual differences in worry and emotionality as components of *trait* test anxiety. In adapting the TAI in different languages, cultures, and age groups, the two-factor structure of the inventory has been consistently verified (Hagtvet, 1976; cf. Spielberger, Gonzalez, Taylor, Algaze, & Anton, 1978; van der Ploeg, Schwarzer, & Spielberger, 1983, 1984, 1985).

Although the heuristic value of the distinction between worry and emotionality as components of test anxiety has been repeatedly demonstrated over the past 20 years, these constructs are not orthogonal; the difference between them is only relative, as Deffenbacher (1980) has observed. Correlations between worry and emotionality reported in the literature vary between .55 and .76. Although we agree with Schwarzer's (1984, p. 206) interpretation of these relations as reflecting both convergent and discriminant validity, in our opinion the theoretical and practical significance of the two-factor interpretation of test anxiety is best justified by the evidence demonstrating that the two components are differentially related to academic performance (criterion validity).

The two-factor structure of Spielberger's (1980) TAI was recently verified in research with the Czech adaptation of the scale (Man & Hosek, 1989); Pearson product–moment correlations between the Worry and Emotionality subscales were .46 for men and .55 for women. For the Czech adaptation, only the Worry subscale correlated significantly with academic performance; these correlations ranged between −.40 and −.51 (Man & Hosek, 1989; Man & Novackova, 1988). In contrast, the correlations between emotionality and academic performance were essentially zero, ranging between −.06 and .05. Similar findings have been reported for the English TAI (Spielberger, 1980).

The major goal of the present study was to investigate the relation between test anxiety, intelligence, and academic performance for Czechoslovakian school boys and girls. Following the procedures used by Schwarzer (1984), we used a simplified form of confirmatory factor analysis to test three hypotheses regarding the relation between worry and emotionality in the factor structure of the Czech TAI. After first reporting the results pertaining to the factor structure of the Czech TAI, the findings with regard to the relationship between test anxiety, intelligence, and academic performance are presented.

METHOD AND PROCEDURE

The research reported in this chapter was carried out in the context of a longitudinal investigation of nonintellectual factors that facilitate or inhibit academic performance. The factor structure of the Czech TAI was evaluated in a study of 153 students (73 boys and 80 girls) who were enrolled in three 7th-grade and three 8th-grade classes in a school located in a small town near Ceské Budejovice, Czechoslovakia. The relationship between test anxiety, ability, and academic achievement was investigated in a study of 75 students (40 boys and 35 girls) from the same school, with an average age of about 14.

The students first completed the 16-item Czech adaptation of the TAI (Man & Hosek, 1989), which was administered to small groups of students with standard instructions. The Czech TAI (TAI-Cz) consisted of 8 worry and 8 emotionality items. After completing the TAI-Cz, the students responded to a Czech adaptation of the Intelligence Structure Test (Amthauer, 1970). Grades in courses on Czech, mathematics, history, and physics were obtained from school records based on the last report of each student's performance. For the statistical analyses, general achievement scores, which ranged from 4 to 20, were derived from the students' grades in the four school subjects.

Confirmatory Factor Analysis

The models for the confirmatory factor analyses, using conventional coding procedures (1 for nonzero estimated parameters; 0 for parameters fixed at zero), were prescribed as follows: Matrix U was restricted to be the diagonal, and, simultaneously, one general factor was hypothesized, with the factor matrix A consisting of a single column with unity loadings. The two-factor hypotheses were evaluated, prescribing A with two columns of nonoverlapping factor loadings for the worry and emotionality items. The possibility of two uncorrelated factors was first tested with P equal to the identity matrix I; the presence of two correlated factors was then tested with P unrestricted. The data were analyzed, taking into account Bentler's delta as a normed index of fit (Bentler & Bonett, 1980).

All three correlation matrices (boys and girls together, boys only, and girls only) were found to differ significantly from I ($p < .01$). Thus, the null hypothesis that the 16 TAI items were uncorrelated in this population was rejected. The COSA model (McDonald, 1978) was then applied, using the least squares (LS) fit function as a first approximation in determining the initial parameter values for maximum likelihood (ML) minimization. The results of the evaluation of the fit of the three alternative models are presented in Table 1. The chi-square tests for the three samples, which varied from 155.1 to 182.2 ($df = 104$), were highly significant ($p < .001$), as can be noted in the first column of Table 1. Thus, the hypothesis of one general factor was clearly inappropriate.

Table 1 Evaluation of Fit of the Three Alternative Test Anxiety Models Specifying One General
Factor, Two Uncorrelated Factors, and Two Correlated Factors

| | | Two factors | |
Correlation matrix	General factor	Uncorrelated	Correlated
Boys and girls			
Chi-square	155	169	107
df	104	104	103
Probability	.00	.00	.28
Delta	.70	.68	.92
RMSR	.07	.11	.01
Boys only			
Chi-square	182	160	118
df	104	104	103
Probability	.00	.00	.11
Delta	.54	.60	.88
RMSR	.08	.13	.03
Girls only			
Chi-square	180	177	116
df	104	104	103
Probability	.00	.00	.15
Delta	.62	.63	.91
RMSR	.08	.14	.02

Note. Delta = Bentler's delta; RMSR = root mean square residual.

Next, the hypothesis that the 16 TAI items clustered into two uncorrelated
Worry and Emotionality factors was tested. The resulting chi-squares, reported in
the middle column of Table 1, were again highly significant for all three samples
($p < .001$). When the hypothesis that these same two factors were correlated was
evaluated, the fit was substantially better, yielding chi-squares with the probability
of .11 for boys, .15 for girls, and .28 for the combined sample. Moreover, the root
mean square residuals (RMSRs) were all .03 or lower. Taken together, these
results strongly support the hypothesis that the TAI consists of two related factors,
Worry and Emotionality. The correlation between these components of test anxiety
was approximately .50.

The final estimations of the A matrices of item factor loadings for the Worry
and Emotionality factors in the three samples are reported in Table 2. As can be
seen, the finding of substantial loadings for each item is consistent with the hypothesis that worry and emotionality are components of test anxiety. The correlations between the factors were .55 for the boys, .68 for the girls, and .69 for the
combined sample. Although these correlations are sizable, the findings are, nevertheless, consistent with the conception of worry and emotionality as independent
(but related) components of test anxiety.

TEST ANXIETY, ABILITY,
AND ACADEMIC PERFORMANCE

The mean achievement scores were 9.80 for boys and 8.37 for the girls (lower
mean, better school achievement). The Pearson correlations of ability with
achievement were .51 for boys and .71 for girls. For the boys, the correlations of

the TAI Total, Worry, and Emotionality scores with achievement were Total, $-.28$; Worry, $-.51$ ($p < .01$); and Emotionality, .04. For the girls, these correlations were Total, $-.24$; Worry, $-.40$ ($p < .01$); and Emotionality, .03.

The correlations of worry and ability with achievement were of about the same magnitude for the boys, although the signs were different. For the girls, intelligence was a better predictor of achievement than worry. Although both worry and TAI Total score predicted academic achievement for both sexes, worry was a much better predictor. The correlations of emotionality with achievement were essentially zero for both sexes.

To examine the interactive effects of test anxiety and ability on academic achievement, the sample was divided into high-ability, low-ability, and test anxiety groups on the basis of the median scores on the ability measure and the Czech TAI Total, Worry, and Emotionality scales. The means and standard deviations of the achievement scores for boys and girls with low or high ability, with scores above or below the median on the TAI Total, Worry, and Emotionality scales, are reported in Table 3. The poorest performers (highest mean scores) were the low-ability, high-emotionality girls and the low-ability, high-worry boys. High worry also had a substantial negative effect on the performance of the high-ability boys and the low-ability girls, whereas high-emotionality scores were associated with better grades for boys, especially those with high ability.

The best grades were achieved by girls with high ability irrespective of their test anxiety level, and by the low-worry, high-ability boys. Indeed, the relation between the three test anxiety measures and academic achievement was negligible for the high-ability girls, whose grades were determined almost entirely by their ability.

To evaluate the Test Anxiety × Ability interactions, several 2 × 2 analyses of variance (ANOVAs) were carried out separately for boys and girls; no significant interactions were found. However, significant main effects were found for boys

Table 2 Item Loadings on the Correlated Worry and Emotionality Factor

Boys and girls		Boys only		Girls only	
Worry	Emotionality	Worry	Emotionality	Worry	Emotionality
.24	—	.49	—	.47	—
.47	—	.51	—	.48	—
.59	—	.53	—	.56	—
.50	—	.47	—	.64	—
.57	—	.50	—	.39	—
.40	—	.73	—	.60	—
.69	—	.65	—	.64	—
.62	—	.46	—	.60	—
—	.43	—	.42	—	.55
—	.62	—	.72	—	.75
—	.55	—	.82	—	.79
—	.41	—	.39	—	.61
—	.54	—	.70	—	.62
—	.45	—	.55	—	.67
—	.68	—	.64	—	.53
—	.22	—	.53	—	.55

Table 3   Means and Standard Deviations for the General Achievement Scores of Students Above and Below the Median in Test Anxiety and Ability

	Boys' ability		Girls' ability	
Test anxiety	Low	High	Low	High
Test Anxiety Inventory total score				
Low				
M	10.20	7.10	8.88	6.67
SD	2.86	3.07	2.10	2.06
High				
M	12.46	9.11	11.78	6.89
SD	2.64	2.93	2.73	2.85
Worry				
Low				
M	9.38	6.58	8.57	6.56
SD	2.56	2.64	2.07	2.19
High				
M	12.62	10.57	11.00	6.63
SD	3.36	2.07	3.38	2.67
Emotionality				
Low				
M	11.82	8.22	9.00	6.57
SD	3.13	2.45	2.77	2.47
High				
M	10.90	7.90	12.80	6.67
SD	3.81	3.38	2.28	2.09

for the TAI Total and Worry measures. Boys with high TAI Total and Worry scores had poorer grades than those with low scores.

A main effect of ability was also consistently found in the ANOVAs. Boys and girls with greater ability scored consistently higher than their less-intelligent counterparts. From these results, it can be concluded that ability is a strong predictor of academic achievement, and that the worry component of test anxiety has the most detrimental effects on performance. This is especially true for boys, regardless of their ability.

DISCUSSION AND CONCLUSIONS

The findings in this investigation of test anxiety, ability, and academic achievement are consistent in some respects with previous research in showing that high test-anxious boys (although not girls) do more poorly in school achievement than their low-anxious counterparts (cf. Hagtvet, 1986; van der Ploeg, 1984). Because no test anxiety–ability interactions were found, our results differ from those reported by van der Ploeg (1984), Sharma and Rao (1983), and Gaudry and Fitzgerald (1971).

The findings of the present study suggest that the interfering effects of test anxiety, and its worry and emotionality components, were not the same for the boys and the girls. However, the degree to which these findings are sample specific or determined by cultural factors is unclear. All of the students were attending an elementary school, which takes 8 years to complete (between the ages of 6 and

14), that is, the students were not streamed. It is generally known that achievement in homogeneous schools is different from achievement at heterogeneous schools (cf. Schwarzer & Schwarzer, 1982).

A possible explanation of the reason that test anxiety appeared to have less influence on the girls in this study is that Czechoslovakian girls are more responsible, careful (painstaking), and willing to exert more effort than Czechoslovakian boys in school activities. Therefore, if they have sufficient preparation time, the anxious girls are more likely to develop effective coping strategies because they are more motivated to do well in school (cf. Krohne, 1987; Krohne & Rogner, 1982).

The standards, strategies, and attributional styles of teachers and parents that produce anxiety, especially evaluation anxiety, were not taken into account in this study (Brophy & Good, 1986; Helmke & Fend, 1982; Krohne, 1980, 1984; Man & Hrabal, in press; Meyer, 1984; van der Poleg, 1984). Because most Western cultures seem to place greater demands on boys, we agree with van der Ploeg's (1984, p. 209) observation that more attention should be given to gender-related differences in parental and teacher attitudes.

SUMMARY

In this study, the Czech adaptation of the Spielberger TAI was administered to elementary school children. The results of a confirmatory factory analysis of the TAI items strongly supported the hypothesis that worry and emotionality are the major substantive components of test anxiety. High test anxiety, and the worry component in particular, was found to have a debilitating effect on academic achievement for boys regardless of their ability and for low-ability girls. The findings were discussed from the perspective of cross-cultural research in terms of cultural factors that may have contributed to sample-specific differences between this study and previous investigations of anxiety, ability, and academic achievement.

REFERENCES

Amthauer, R. (1970). *Intelligenz-Struktur-Test (IST-70) [Intelligence Structure Test]*. Göttingen, Federal Republic of Germany: Hogrefe.

Bentler, P. M., & Bonett, D. G. (1980). Significance tests and goodness of fit in the analysis of covariance structures. *Psychological Bulletin, 88*, 588–606.

Bowler, R. (1982). A brief review of test anxiety in West German schools. In R. Schwarzer, H. M. van der Ploeg, C. D. Spielberger (Eds.), *Advances in test anxiety research* (Vol. 1, pp. 85–94). Lisse, the Netherlands: Swets & Zeitlinger/Erlbaum.

Brophy, J., & Good, T. L. (1986). Teacher behavior and student achievement. In M. C. Wittrock (Ed.), *Handbook of research on teaching* (3rd ed. pp. 328–375). New York: Macmillan.

Deffenbacher, J. L. (1980). Worry and emotionality in test anxiety. In I. G. Sarason (Ed.), *Test anxiety: Theory, research, and applications* (pp. 111–128). Hillsdale, NJ: Erlbaum.

Gaudry, E., & Fitzgerald, D. (1971). Test anxiety, intelligence and academic achievement. In E. Gaudry & C. D. Spielberger (Eds.), *Anxiety and educational achievement* (pp. 155–162). New York: Wiley.

Gjesme, T. (1972). Sex differences in the relationship between test anxiety and school performance. *Psychological Report, 30*, 907–914.

Hagtvet, K. A. (1976). Worry and emotionality components of test anxiety in different sex and age groups of elementary school children. *Psychological Reports, 39*, 1327–1334.

Hagtvet, K. A. (1986, April). *Interaction of anxiety and ability on academic achievement: A simultaneous consideration of parameters*. Prepared for International Symposium on Test Anxiety, AERA annual meeting, San Francisco.

Heckhausen, H. (1982). Task-irrelevant cognitions during an exam: Incidence and effects. In H. W. Krohne & L. Laux (Eds.), *Achievement, stress, and anxiety* (pp. 247–274). Washington, DC: Hemisphere.

Heinrich, D. L. (1979). The causal influence of anxiety on academic achievement for students of differing intellectual ability. *Applied Psychological Measurement, 3,* 351–359.

Helmke, A., & Fend, H. (1982). Diagnostic sensitivity of teachers and parents with respect to the test anxiety of students. In R. Schwarzer, H. M. van der Ploeg, & C. D. Spielberger (Eds.), *Advances in test anxiety research* (Vol. 1, pp. 115–128). Lisse, the Netherlands: Swets & Zeitlinger/Erlbaum.

Hodapp, V., Laux, L., & Spielberger, C. D. (1982). Theorie und Messung der emotionalen und kognitiven Komponente der Prüfungsangst. [Theory and measurement of emotional and cognitive components of test anxiety]. *Zeitschift für Differentielle und Diagnostische Psychologie, 3,* 169–184.

Jerusalem, M. (1985). A longitudinal field study with trait worry and trait emotionality: Methodological problems. In H. M. van der Ploeg, R. Schwarzer, & C. D. Spielberger (Eds.), *Advances in test anxiety research* (Vol. 4, pp. 23–24). Lisse, the Netherlands: Swets & Zeitlinger/Erlbaum.

Krohne, H. W. (1980). Prüfungstangst: Defensive motivation in selbstwertrelevanten situationen. [Test anxiety: Defensive motivation in self-evaluation situations]. *Unterrichtswissenschaft, 8,* 226–242.

Krohne, H. W. (1984). Analysen der structur der erziehungsstil—inventars [Analysis of structure of child rearing inventory]. Mainzer Berichtezur Personlichkeitsforschung (Nr.4) University of Mainz: Scientific report.

Krohne, H. W. (1987). Coping research: Current theoretical and methodological developments. *Mainzer Berichte zur Persönlichkeitsforschung* (Nr. 15).

Krohne, H. W., & Rogner, J. (1982). Repression-sensitization as a central construct in coping research. In H. M. Krohne & L. Laux (Eds.), *Achievement, stress, and anxiety* (pp. 187–193). Washington, DC: Hemisphere.

Liebert, R. M., & Morris, L. W. (1967). Cognitive and emotional components of test anxiety: A distinction and some initial data. *Psychological Reports, 20,* 975–978.

Man, F., & Hosek, V. (1989). The development and validation of the Czech form of the Test Anxiety Inventory. In R. Schwarzer, H. M. van der Ploeg, & C. D. Spielberger (Eds.), *Advances in test anxiety research* (Vol. 6, pp. 233–243). Lisse, the Netherlands: Swets & Zeitlinger.

Man, F., & Hrabal, V., Jr. (in press). Self-concept of ability, social consequences anxiety, and attribution as correlates of action control. In F. Halisch & H. L. van den Bercken (Eds.). *International perspectives on achievement and task motivation.* Lisse, the Netherlands: Swets & Zeitlinger.

Man, F., & Novackova, I. (1988, July). *The relationship among academic performance, test anxiety, intelligence and sex.* Paper presented at the 9th International STAR Conference, Padua, Italy.

McDonald, R. P. (1978). A simple comprehensive model for the analysis of covariance structures. *British Journal of Mathematical Statistical Psychology, 31,* 59–72.

Meyer, W. U. (1984). *Das Konzept von der eigenen Begabung.* [Self-concept of ability]. Bern, Switzerland: Huber.

Morris, L. W., Davis, M. A., & Hutchings, C. J. (1981). Cognitive and emotional components of anxiety: Literature review and a revised worry-emotionality scale. *Journal of Educational Psychology, 73,* 541–555.

Sarason, I. G. (1975). Anxiety and self-preoccupation. In I. G. Sarason & C. D. Spielberger (Eds.), *Stress and anxiety* (Vol. 2, pp. 27–44). New York: Wiley.

Schwarzer, R. (1975). *Schulangst und Lernerfolg. Eur Diagnose und zur Bedeutung von Leistungsangst in der Schule.* [Test anxiety and school success. To diagnose from the viewpoint of school anxiety]. Dusseldorf, Federal Republic of Germany: Schwann.

Schwarzer, R. (1984). Worry and emotionality as separate components in test anxiety. *International Review of Applied Psychology, 33,* 205–219.

Schwarzer, R., Jerusalem, M., & Lange, B. (1982). A longitudinal study of worry and emotionality in German secondary school children. In R. Schwarzer, H. M. van der Ploeg, & C. D. Spielberger (Eds.), *Advances in test anxiety research* (Vol. 1, pp. 67–81). Lisse, the Netherlands: Swets & Zeitlinger/Erlbaum.

Schwarzer, R., & Schwarzer, C. (1982). Test anxiety with respect to school reference groups. In R. Schwarzer, H. M. van der Ploeg, & C. D. Spielberger (Eds.), *Advances in test anxiety research* (Vol. 1, pp. 95–104). Lisse, the Netherlands: Swets & Zeitlinger/Erlbaum.

Schwarzer, R., Van der Ploeg, & Spielberger, C. D. (Eds.). (1989). Advances in test anxiety research (vol. 6). Lisse, the Netherlands: Swets & Zeitlinger.

Sharma, S., & Rao, U. (1983). Academic performance in different school courses as related to self-acceptance, test anxiety, and intelligence. In H. M. van der Ploeg, R. Schwarzer, & C. D. Spielberger (Eds.), *Advances in test anxiety research* (Vol. 2, pp. 111–118). Lisse, the Netherlands: Swets & Zeitlinger/Erlbaum.

Sipos, K., Sipos, M., & Spielberger, C. D. (1985). The development and validation of the Hungarian form of the Test Anxiety Inventory. In H. M. van der Ploeg, R. Schwarzer, & C. D. Spielberger (Eds.), *Advances in test anxiety research* (Vol. 4, pp. 221–228). Lisse, the Netherlands: Swets & Zeitlinger.

Spielberger, C. D. (1962). The effects of manifest anxiety on the academic achievement of college students. *Mental Hygiene, 46,* 420–426.

Spielberger, C. D. (1972). Conceptual and methodological issues in anxiety research. In C. D. Spielberger (Ed.), *Anxiety: Current trends in theory and research* (Vol. 2, pp. 487–493). New York: Academic Press.

Spielberger, C. D. (1980). *Manual for the Test Anxiety Inventory.* Palo Alto, CA: Consulting Psychologists Press.

Spielberger, C. D., Gonzalez, H. P., Taylor, C. J., Algaze, B., & Anton, W. D. (1978). Examination stress and test anxiety. In C. D. Spielberger and I. G. Sarason (Eds.), *Stress and anxiety* (Vol. 5, 167–191). New York: Wiley.

Van der Ploeg, H. M. (1982). The relationship of worry and emotionality to performance in Dutch school children. In R. Schwarzer, H. M. van der Ploeg, & C. D. Spielberger (Eds.), *Advances in test anxiety research* (Vol. 1, pp. 55–66). Lisse, the Netherlands: Swets & Zeitlinger.

Van der Ploeg, H. M. (1983). The validation of the Dutch form of the Test Anxiety Inventory. In H. M. van der Ploeg, R. Schwarzer, & C. D. Spielberger (Eds.), *Advances in test anxiety research* (Vol. 2, pp. 191–202). Lisse, the Netherlands: Swets & Zeitlinger/Erlbaum.

Van der Ploeg, H. M. (1984). Worry, emotionality, intelligence, and academic performance in male and female Dutch secondary school children. In H. M. van der Ploeg, R. Schwarzer, & C. D. Spielberger (Eds.), *Advances in test anxiety research* (Vol. 3, pp. 201–210). Lisse, the Netherlands: Swets & Zeitlinger/Erlbaum.

Van der Ploeg, H. M., Schwarzer, R., & Spielberger, C. D. (Eds.). (1983). *Advances in test anxiety research* (Vol. 2). Lisse, the Netherlands: Swets & Zeitlinger/Erlbaum.

Van der Ploeg, H. M., Schwarzer, R., & Spielberger, C. D. (Eds.). (1984). *Advances in test anxiety research* (Vol. 3). Lisse, the Netherlands: Swets & Zeitlinger.

Van der Ploeg, H. M., Schwarzer, R., & Spielberger, C. D. (Eds.). (1985). *Advances in test anxiety research* (Vol. 4). Lisse, the Netherlands: Swets & Zeitlinger.

Wine, J. D. (1982). Evaluation anxiety: A cognitive-attentional construct. In H. S. Krohne & L. Laux (Eds.), *Achievement, stress, and anxiety* (pp. 207–219). Washington, DC: Hemisphere.

16

Assessment of Anxiety
in Spanish Elementary School Children

Domingo E. Gómez-Fernández
University of Santiago de Compostela, Spain

Charles D. Spielberger
University of South Florida, USA

Psychologists, psychiatrists, and other mental health professionals have often reported that they lack valid measures for evaluating prevention strategies and treatment programs aimed at reducing children's anxiety (Gómez-Fernández & Pulido-Picouto, 1989). Administrators, educators, and clinicians have also recognized the importance of the early identification of children who are prone to experience intense levels of anxiety, because such children are often characterized by a high incidence of drug use, as well as antisocial behaviors (Gómez-Fernández, 1981a, 1981b). Consequently, the development of valid and reliable measures for assessing anxiety in children constitutes an especially important challenge for psychologists concerned with mental health and personality assessment.

In recent years, increasing interest in the assessment of anxiety has stimulated the construction of numerous scales, checklists, and inventories. Indeed, in the evaluation of anxiety clinicians and researchers seem to have literally endorsed Binet and Simon's (1973, p. 329) dictum with regard to measuring intelligence: "It matters very little what the tests are so long as they are numerous."

Of the numerous scales for measuring anxiety that are currently available, the State–Trait Anxiety Inventory (STAI; Spielberger, 1983; Spielberger, Gorsuch, & Lushene, 1970) has been used more often than any other instrument. Since its publication in 1970, the STAI has been translated or adapted in 41 languages and dialects (see Spielberger, 1989), and various forms of the scale, including the Spanish adaptation (Spielberger, González, Martínez, Natalicio, & Natalicio, 1971) and the State–Trait Anxiety Inventory for Children (STAIC; Spielberger, Edwards, Lushene, Montuori, & Platzek, 1973), have been used to assess anxiety in more than 3,000 studies (Spielberger, 1989).

This research was supported in part by a grant from the Spanish Ministry of Education (*Dirección General de Investigación Científica y Tecnica*). The authors would like to express their appreciation to Yolanda C. León, Richard Rickman, and Virginia Berch for their assistance in the analysis of the data and the preparation of the manuscript.

This chapter was prepared while Professor Gómez-Fernández was Visiting Professor at the Center for Research in Behavioral Medicine and Health Psychology, University of South Florida, Tampa, Florida.

The main goal of the study presented in this chapter was to examine the reliability and psychometric properties of the *Inventario de Ansiedad Rasgo Estado para Niños* (IDAREN; Bauermeister, Forastieri, & Spielberger, 1976; Bauermeister, Fumero, Villamil-Forastieri, & Spielberger, 1986), the Spanish version of the STAIC. Although the STAIC is one of the most widely used and easily administered measures of children's anxiety, relatively few studies have investigated the psychometric characteristics of this scale in cross-cultural research. A second goal of this study was to report evidence of the concurrent validity and the factor structure of the IDAREN, based on data collected with Spanish elementary school children. Finally, the state and trait anxiety scores of children from Spain, Puerto Rico, and the United States are compared.

METHOD

Subjects

The participants in this study were 183 third-grade elementary school children (122 boys and 61 girls) enrolled in six different schools in the provinces of La Coruna, Lugo, Orense, and Pontevedra in the region of Galicia, Spain. Approximately 80% of the population in this region speak Galician as their mother tongue, 7% speak Castilian, and 13% are "balanced" bilinguals who are equally fluent in both languages. The linguistic background of the sample is further complicated by the fact that approximately 12% of the participants were children of first-generation immigrants.

Test Instruments and Procedure

The IDAREN, the Child Anxiety Scale (CAS), and the Eysenck Personality Questionnaire—Junior (EPQ-J) were administered with standard instructions by the investigators, who were assisted by classroom teachers. The children were tested during regular class periods in groups of 20–25 pupils. The CAS was administered first, followed by the EPQ-J and the IDAREN Trait (T-Anxiety) and State (S-Anxiety) scales. Scores for each child were calculated for all four measures.

The IDAREN was developed by Bauermeister et al. (1976) and consists of 20 S-Anxiety and 20 T-Anxiety items. The instructions for the IDAREN S-Anxiety Scale require children to respond to each item by circling a word or phrase that best describes the *intensity* of their feelings of anxiety at a particular time (e.g., "very frightened," "frightened," "not frightened"). The IDAREN T-Anxiety Scale requires children to indicate how they generally feel. In responding to each T-Anxiety item (e.g., "My hands get sweaty"), children report how often they have experienced the particular symptom of anxiety by rating themselves on the following 3-point Frequency scale: "hardly ever," "sometimes," and "often."

The CAS consists of 20 true–false items designed to measure general anxiety in children (Gillis, 1980). The CAS was derived from the Early School Personality Questionnaire (ESPQ; Coan & Cattell, 1966) by successive factor analyses of the intercorrelations among the 320 ESPQ items. A Spanish adaptation of the CAS was recently developed by Gómez-Fernández and Pulido-Picouto (1989).

The EPQ-J (S. B. G. Eysenck, 1965) consists of 81 true–false items that yield measures of the following five personality dimensions: neuroticism, extraversion, psychoticism, sociability, and antisocial behavior (S. B. G. Eysenck, 1965). It was derived from the Eysenck Personality Inventory (EPI; H. J. Eysenck & Eysenck, 1964), which measures the same characteristics in adults. Only the findings for the EPQ-J Neuroticism (N) Scale are reported in this chapter.

RESULTS

The means, standard deviations, and alpha reliability coefficients of the IDAREN scales for the Spanish third-grade children are presented in Table 1. Note that the mean T-Anxiety scores for the boys and girls were almost the same. Although the S-Anxiety scores of the girls were slightly higher than those of the boys, this difference was not statistically significant.

Alpha coefficients for the IDAREN T-Anxiety and S-Anxiety scales were computed by using the Kuder–Richardson 20 as modified by Chronbach (1951). The alphas for the T-Anxiety Scale were .75 for the boys and .85 for the girls; the S-Anxiety alphas for boys and girls were .78 and .87, respectively. Further evidence of the internal consistency of the IDAREN was reflected in the median item-remainder correlations of .33 for the T-Anxiety items and .40 for the S-Anxiety items. Similar item-remainder correlations have been reported for the IDAREN for children in Puerto Rico (Bauermeister et al., 1986) and for the STAIC for American children (Spielberger et al., 1973).

Because there were no significant differences between the S-Anxiety and T-Anxiety scores of boys and girls, the data for the two groups were combined in order to provide more stable percentile ranks for the total sample. The T-Anxiety and S-Anxiety raw scores and percentile ranks for boys and girls are presented in Table 2. The median T-Anxiety and S-Anxiety scores for the total sample were approximately 31 and 30, respectively, as can be noted in Table 2.

The correlations between the IDAREN S-Anxiety and T-Anxiety scales were .05 for the boys and .13 for the girls. Correlations between the STAIC S-Anxiety and T-Anxiety scales reported by Montuori (1971) for fifth- and sixth-grade American boys and girls ranged between − .05 and .31, with a median correlation of .13. Somewhat higher STAIC state–trait correlations for fourth-, fifth-, and sixth-grade

Table 1 Means, Standard Deviations, and Reliability Measures of the *Inventario de Ansiedad Rasgo Estado para Niños* T-Anxiety and S-Anxiety Scales for Spanish Children

Scale	Boys (n = 122)	Girls (n = 61)	t
T-Anxiety			
M	44.41	44.00	0.70
SD	3.64	4.10	
Alpha	.75	.85	
S-Anxiety			
M	35.26	36.32	− 1.14
SD	5.99	5.61	
Alpha	.78	.87	

Table 2 Inventario de Ansiedad Rasgo Estado para Niños Raw
Scores and Percentile Ranks for Spanish Children

Raw score	T-Anxiety	S-Anxiety
49–60	99	99
47	98	99
46	96	99
44	92	98
43	88	97
42	86	96
41	84	95
40	81	94
39	78	90
37	73	87
36	66	85
35	57	81
32	55	75
31	49	64
30	43	51
29	35	46
28	29	42
27	24	34
26	20	24
25	14	20
24	11	13
23	8	10
22	5	7
21	1	4
20	1	1

American children have been reported by Edwards (1972). These ranged from .11 to .50.

Correlations obtained between the IDAREN T-Anxiety Scale and the CAS and EPQ-J N Scale scores provide evidence of the concurrent validity. For the total sample, the IDAREN T-Anxiety Scale correlated .37 with the CAS and .31 with the EPQ-J N Scale. Montuori (1971) reported a correlation of .63 between the STAIC T-Anxiety Scale and the Children's Manifest Anxiety Scale.

Factor Structure of the IDAREN

The scores for the 40 IDAREN items were factor analyzed, using the principal-components method. Four factors with eigenvalues greater than unity were identified. Cattell's (1966) scree test also suggested that four factors should be extracted, but the resulting three- and four-factor solutions were lacking in simple structure. In terms of simple structure, the best solution was achieved when two factors were rotated by the varimax procedure (Nie, 1975).

The salient item loadings for the two-factor solution are reported in Table 3. Of the 20 trait items (numbered 1–20), 14 had salient loadings (.30 or higher) on Factor 1. Only one T-Anxiety item (Item 19) had a salient loading on Factor 2, but this item also had a loading of approximately the same magnitude on Factor 1. The dominant loading for 12 of the 20 S-Anxiety items (Items 21–40) was on Factor 2, whereas 8 S-Anxiety items had higher loadings on Factor 1 than on Factor 2.

The finding that 9 S-Anxiety items had salient loadings (.30 or higher) on

Factor 1 was surprising and problematic. As can be noted in Table 3, 8 of these were anxiety-absent items (e.g., calm, pleasant, satisfied, happy, sure, good, nice, and cheerful). Moreover, 8 of the 9 items with strong loadings (.40 or higher) on Factor 2 were anxiety-present items (e.g., upset, nervous, scared, worried, frightened, troubled, bothered, and terrified). Thus, Factor 1 was defined primarily by T-Anxiety items, but also included S-Anxiety-absent items, whereas Factor 2 consisted almost entirely of S-Anxiety-present items.

Table 3 Item Loadings for the Two-Factor Solution of the 40 *Inventario de Ansiedad Rasgo Estado para Niños* Items

		Loading	
Item		Factor 1: Trait anxiety	Factor 2: State anxiety
1.	I worry about making mistakes.	.58	
2.	I feel like crying.	.43	
3.	I feel unhappy.		(.23)
4.	I have trouble making up my mind.	(.27)	
5.	Difficult to face my problems.		(.21)
6.	I worry too much.	.39	
7.	I get upset at home.	(.21)	
8.	I am shy.	.32	
9.	I feel troubled.	.44	
10.	Unimportant thoughts . . . bother me.	.41	
11.	I worry about school.	.47	
12.	I have trouble deciding what to do.	.36	
13.	My heart beats fast.		(.19)
14.	I am secretly afraid.	.51	
15.	I worry about my parents.	(.27)	
16.	My hands get sweaty.	.45	
17.	I worry about things that may happen.	.31	
18.	It is hard for me to fall asleep at night.	.39	
19.	I get a funny feeling in my stomach.	.32	−.32
20.	I worry about what others think of me.	.37	
21.	I feel calm.	.31	.30
22.	I feel upset.		.46
23.	I feel pleasant.	.41	(−.23)
24.	I feel nervous.		.53
25.	I feel jittery.		(.25)
26.	I feel rested.		.31
27.	I feel scared.		.56
28.	I feel relaxed.		.35
29.	I feel worried.		.54
30.	I feel satisfied.	.36	
31.	I feel frightened.		.72
32.	I feel happy.	.48	
33.	I feel sure.	.46	
34.	I feel good.	.36	(−.21)
35.	I feel troubled.		.57
36.	I feel bothered.		.57
37.	I feel nice.	.30	−.44
38.	I feel terrified.		.62
39.	I feel mixed up.		(.27)
40.	I feel cheerful.	.31	(−.21)
Eigenvalue		5.34	2.72

Note. Only salient loadings above .30 are reported, except for items that had no salient loadings, for which the highest loadings are indicated in parentheses.

As Factor 1 in this study consisted primarily of trait items and Factor 2 consisted primarily of state items, these findings provide further empirical evidence of the importance of the distinction between trait and state anxiety. Moreover, the IDAREN factors identified for the Spanish children in this study are similar to the results that have been reported for the English form of the STAI (e.g., Gaudry & Poole, 1975; Vagg, Spielberger, & O'Hearn, 1980).

Cluster Analysis of the IDAREN

To further clarify the structure of the IDAREN, separate cluster analyses were carried out for the T-Anxiety and S-Anxiety items, using the BMDP1 cluster program (Dixon, 1973), which uses Ward's method and squared Euclidean distance as the distance measure. The dendogram for the T-Anxiety items is presented in Figure 1. Only one T-Anxiety cluster was identified; it contained 10 items with an attained distance (similarity) of 29.9. The remaining 10 T-Anxiety items were individually connected with this single cluster, but the similarity was relatively low. Although consisting mainly of "worry" items (1, 18, 12, 11, 15, 17), the T-Anxiety cluster also included a subcluster of three closely related items (14, 16, 19) that reflected emotionality (afraid, sweaty, and funny feeling in my stomach).

The cluster dendogram for the IDAREN S-Anxiety items, presented in Figure 2, appears to identify two distinct clusters. The first cluster was defined by eight items (21, 23, 32, 34, 40, 33, 37, 30) with content that reflected the absence of anxiety; therefore, this cluster was labeled *anxiety absent*. The second cluster, consisting of 9 items (22, 24, 27, 31, 38, 35, 29, 36, 39) that described symptoms of anxiety, was labeled *anxiety present*. Three items (28, 25, 26) that were not closely related to either cluster seemed to reflect relaxed or excited motoric states rather than anxiety feelings or cognitions.

The means, standard deviations, and alpha coefficients of the IDAREN T-Anxiety and S-Anxiety scales for the Spanish children in the present study are compared in Table 4 with the IDAREN and STAIC scores of Puerto Rican and American children. The mean T-Anxiety scores of the boys and girls in each of the three samples were quite similar, but the mean scores for the Spanish children of both sexes were substantially higher than those of the other groups. The T-Anxiety scores of the American children were higher that those of the Puerto Rican children.

The IDAREN mean S-Anxiety scores of the boys and girls in each country were similar, but the S-Anxiety means of the Spanish children were somewhat higher than those of the other groups. The American children had the lowest S-Anxiety scores. For the Spanish and American children, the S-Anxiety scores for both boys and girls were substantially lower than the corresponding T-Anxiety scores for these groups, whereas the S-Anxiety scores of the Puerto Rican children were higher than their corresponding T-Anxiety scores.

DISCUSSION

The internal consistency reliability of the IDAREN in the present study was generally satisfactory for both sexes, as indicted by T-Anxiety alpha coefficients of .75 for boys and .85 for girls, and S-Anxiety alphas of .78 for boys and .87 for girls. The lower alpha coefficients of the boys may indicate that they experienced

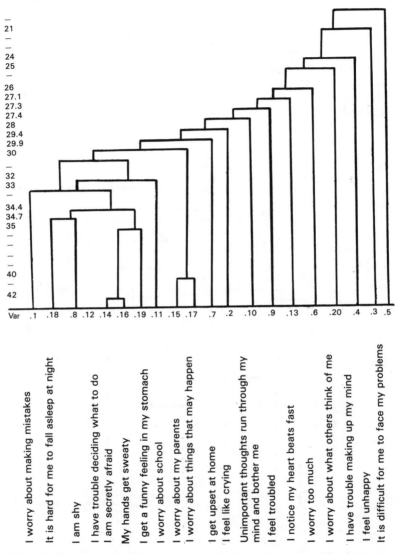

Figure 1 Cluster analysis of *Inventario de Ansiedad Rasgo Estado para Niños* (T-Anxiety).

more difficulty than the girls in responding to the IDAREN. From a cross-cultural perspective, the findings of the present study indicated that the internal consistency reliability of the IDAREN for children in Spain was comparable to that of the IDAREN for the children in Puerto Rico (Bauermeister et al., 1976) and the STAIC for American children (Spielberger et al., 1973).

Evidence of the concurrent validity of the IDAREN in this study was supported by the moderate correlations with the CAS (r = .37) and the EPQ-J N Scale (r =

.31). On the assumption that the IDAREN and the CAS both measure trait anxiety, higher correlations between these scales were expected. It should be noted, however, that Gillis (1980) failed to report any evidence of the concurrent validity of the CAS. Only a moderate correlation between the EPQ-J N Scale and the IDAREN was expected because the concept of neurosis is considerably broader than that of anxiety (Cattell & Scheier, 1961; H. J. Eysenck, 1969; Scheier, 1972).

When all 40 IDAREN items were factored together, separate trait and state anxiety factors were identified. The results of the factor analysis were quite similar to those obtained with the original English version of the STAIC (Spielberger et al., 1973) and to the findings of a number of investigators with the STAI (Bernstein &

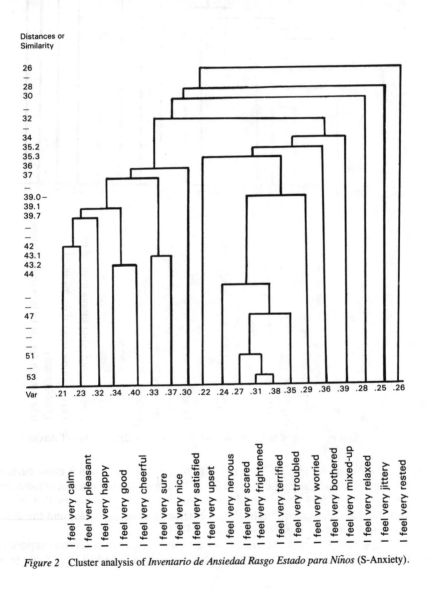

Figure 2 Cluster analysis of *Inventario de Ansiedad Rasgo Estado para Niños* (S-Anxiety).

Table 4 Means, Standard Deviations, and Alpha Reliability for the *Inventario de Ansiedad Rasgo Estado para Niños* and State–Trait Anxiety Inventory for Children Scores of Spanish, Puerto Rican, and American Children

Scale	Spanish[a]		Puerto Rican[b]		American[c]	
	Boys (n = 122)	Girls (n = 61)	Boys (n = 115)	Girls (n = 117)	Boys (n = 817)	Girls (n = 737)
T-Anxiety						
M	44.4	44.0	29.1	29.8	36.7	38.0
SD	3.64	4.10	4.97	5.93	6.32	5.71
Alpha	.75	.85	.80	.84	.84	.79
S-Anxiety						
M	35.2	36.3	33.1	34.3	31.0	30.7
SD	5.99	5.61	6.12	6.91	6.68	6.01
Alpha	.78	.87	.83	.86	.70	.74

[a]Gómez-Fernández & Pulido-Picouto (1989)
[b]Bauermeister et al. (1976)
[c]Spielberger et al. (1973)

Eveland, 1982; Vagg et al., 1980). To further clarify the nature of the IDAREN's factor structure, the trait and state items were evaluated in separate cluster analyses. For the T-Anxiety Scale, only one cluster was identified, containing 10 of the 20 T-Anxiety items. For the IDAREN S-Anxiety Scale, two distinct clusters were identified, one consisting primarily of the 12 anxiety-present items and the other consisting of the 8 anxiety-absent items. Other investigators (Shek, 1988; Sherwood & Westerback, 1983; Vagg et al., 1980), have also identified anxiety-present and anxiety-absent S-Anxiety factors in previous research.

The Galician Spanish children in the present study scored higher in T-Anxiety than the American children and much higher than the Puerto Rican children. The mean S-Anxiety scores of the Spanish children were also somewhat higher than those of the Puerto Rican and the American children. The higher anxiety scores of the Spanish Galician children in this study were consistent with previous research (Gómez-Fernández, 1981a, 1981b; Pulido-Picouto, 1986) and appear to reflect the psychosocial consequences of the bilinguism problem in the educational system of Galicia.

A number of children in this study were first-generation immigrants living abroad with their grandparents, and without their fathers' affective and very necessary contact. These conditions appeared to foster negative attitudes toward the host culture and its values, including negative classroom attitudes that inhibit learning (Fillmore, 1979). The findings of higher anxiety scores for the Spanish children seemed to reflect these attitudes and support "the impression that a man alters his personality when speaking another language" (Lowie, 1945, p. 249). Lewis (1981) has suggested that high anxiety reflects the psychological disturbances resulting from irregular transfer from one language to another, the way the two languages were acquired, and the attitudes of parents and teachers.

The findings of the present study indicate that the IDAREN shows considerable promise for use by educators, investigators, and clinicians in cross-cultural research on children's anxiety in Spanish-speaking countries. Future research with the IDAREN should be aimed at determining the reliability of the inventory for measuring anxiety in children from other Hispanic cultures.

SUMMARY

The results of the present study provide evidence of the reliability and concurrent validity of the IDAREN, the Spanish version of the STAIC. The reliability of the IDAREN for Spanish elementary school children in Galicia was comparable to that found for the IDAREN with Puerto Rican children and for the STAIC with American children. Concurrent validity was demonstrated by moderate correlations between the IDAREN and the CAS and somewhat lower correlations with the N Scale of the EPQ-J.

Factor analysis of all 40 IDAREN items identified two main factors: State Anxiety and Trait Anxiety. Separate cluster analyses for the T-Anxiety and S-Anxiety items revealed a single T-Anxiety cluster, comprising largely worry items and two distinctive S-Anxiety clusters that consisted of anxiety-present and anxiety-absent items. Spanish children had higher state and trait anxiety scores than their Puerto Rican and American counterparts, which was attributed to the stress of residing in a bilingual culture, especially for children of first-generation immigrants.

REFERENCES

Bauermeister, J. J., Forastieri, B. V., & Spielberger, C. D. (1976). Development and validation of the Spanish form of the State–Trait Anxiety Inventory for Children (STAIC). In C. D. Spielberger & R. Diaz-Guerrero (Eds.), *Cross-cultural anxiety* (Vol. 1, 69–85). Washington, DC: Hemisphere/Wiley.

Bauermeister, J. J., Fumero, D. C., Villamil-Forestieri, B., & Spielberger, C. D. (1986). Confiabilidad y validez del inventario de ansiedad rasgo-estado para niños puertoriquenos y panamenos [Reliability and validity of the IDAREN]. *Revista Interamericana de Psicolgia, 20,* 1–20.

Bernstein, I. H., & Eveland, D. C. (1982). State vs trait anxiety: A case study in confirmatory factor analysis. *Personality and Individual Differences, 3,* 361–372.

Binet, A., & Simon, T. (1973). *The development of intelligence in children.* New York: Arno Press. (Original published 1911)

Cattell, R. B. (1966). Anxiety and motivation: Theory and crucial experiments. In C. D. Spielberger (Ed.), *Anxiety and behavior* (Vol. 1, 23–62). New York: Academic Press.

Cattell, R. B., & Scheier, I. H. (1961). *The meaning and measurement of neuroticism and anxiety.* New York: Wiley.

Coan, R. W., & Cattell, R. B. (1966). *Early School Personality Questionnaire.* Champaign, IL: Institute for Personality and Ability Testing.

Cronbach, L. J. (1951). Coefficient alpha and the internal structure of tests. *Psychometrica, 16,* 297–335.

Dixon, W. J. (1973). *BMD biomedical computer programs.* Berkeley: University of California Press.

Edwards, C. D. (1972). *Stress in the schools: A study of anxiety and self-esteem in Black and White elementary school children.* Unpublished doctoral dissertation, Florida State University.

Eysenck, H. J. (1969). *Personality structure and measurement.* San Diego, CA: Knapp.

Eysenck, H. J., & Eysenck, S. B. G. (1964). *Manual of the Eysenck Personality Inventory.* London: Hodder Stoughton.

Eysenck, S. B. G. (1965). *Manual of the Junior Eysenck Personality Inventory.* London: University Press.

Fillmore, L. W. (1979). Individual differences in second language acquisition. In C. J Fillmore, D. Kempler, & W. Wang (Eds.), *Individual differences in language ability and language behaviour* (pp. 203–229). New York: Academic Press.

Gaudry, E., & Poole, C. (1975). A further validation of the state–trait distinction in anxiety research. *Multivariate Behavioral Research, 10,* 331–341.

Gillis, J. S. (1980). *Manual for the Child Anxiety Scale*. Champaign, IL: Institute for Personality and Ability Testing.

Gómez-Fernández, D. E. (1981a). *Analisis y evaluación de la personalidad infantil a traves de la adaptacion espanola del ESPQ*. [*The analysis and assessment of the early personality by the Spanish version of ESPQ*]. Unpublished doctoral dissertation, University Complutense of Madrid.

Gómez-Fernández, D. E. (1981b). El ESPQ, un neuvo cuestionario de personalidad infantil a disposicion de la población infantil Espanola [The ESPQ: A new questionnaire to evaluate Spanish infant school children]. *Revista de Psicologia General y Aplicada, 36*, 451–472.

Gómez-Fernández, D. E., & Pulido-Picouto, M. T. (1989). *Cuestionario de Ansiedad Infantil [Manual for the Spanish version of CAS]*. Madrid, Spain: TEA Ediciones.

Lewis, E. G. *(1981)*. *Bilingualism and bilinqual education*. *Oxford: Pergamon Press*.

Lowie, R. *(1945)*. *A case of bilinguilism*. *Word, 1*, 249–259.

Montuori, T. T. (1971). *The effects of stress and anxiety verbal conditioning in children*. Unpublished doctoral dissertation, Florida State University.

Nie, N. H., Hull, C. H., Jenkins, J. G., Steinbrenner, K., & Bent, D. H. (1975). Statistical package for the social sciences. New York: McGraw-Hill.

Pulido-Picouto, M. T. (1986). *Analisis y evaluacion de la ansiedad infantil a traves de respuestas emitidas por escolares gallegos a la escala de ansiedad CAS-Gillis [The assessment of child anxiety from the Spanish version of CAS]*. Unpublished master's thesis, University of Santiago de Compostela (Spain).

Scheier, I.H. (1972). Anxiety at a distance. In R. M. Dreger (Ed.), *Multivariate personality research* (pp. 327–351). Baton Rouge: Claitor.

Shek, D. T. L. (1988). Reliability and Factorial structure of the Chinese version of the State–Trait Anxiety Inventory. *Journal of Psychopathology and Behavioral Assessment, 10*, 303–317.

Sherwood, R. D., & Westerback, M. E. (1983). A factor analytic study of the State–Trait Anxiety Inventory utilized with pre-service elementary teachers. *Journal of Research in Science Teaching, 20*, 225–229.

Spielberger, C. D. (1983). Manual for the State–Trait Anxiety Inventory. Palo Alto, CA: Consulting Psychologists Press.

Spielberger, C. D. (1989). *State–Trait Anxiety Inventory: A comprehensive bibliography*. Palo Alto, CA: Consulting Psychologists Press.

Spielberger, C. D., Edwards, C. D., Lushene, R. E., Montuori, J., & Platzek, D. (1973). *State-Trait Anxiety Inventory for Children (STAIC): Preliminary Manual*. Palo Alto, CA: Consulting Psychologists Press.

Spielberger, C. D., González, H. P., Martínez, A., Natalicio, L. F., & Natalicio, D. S. (1971). Development of the Spanish edition of the State–Trait Anxiety Inventory. *Interamerican Journal of Psychology, 5*, 145–158.

Spielberger, C. D., Gorsuch, R. C., & Lushene, R. F. (1970). *Manual for the State-Trait Anxiety Inventory*. Palo Alto, CA: Consulting Psychologists Press.

Vagg, P. R., Spielberger, C. D., & O'Hearn, T. P. (1980). Is the State–Trait Anxiety Inventory multidimensional? *Personality and Individual Differences, 1*, 207–214.

Author Index

Subject Index